"Cancer survivor Yvonne Ortega has written a wonderfully honest and uplifting book. Those who walk through the valley of the shadow of cancer no longer have to travel alone. They have Yvonne to walk through it, hand in hand, with them."

Donna Partow, author, *Becoming the Woman I Want to Be*

"Yvonne Ortega's honesty will create a bond with readers and encourage them to face their own pain and fear armed with the 'Hope Builders' from God's Word that sustained her. This is must reading for anyone diagnosed with cancer as well as for their family and friends."

Marlene Bagnull, author, *My Turn to Care*

"This book can help women as they go through their experience with cancer, but it's equally helpful for families and caregivers."

Cecil Murphey, coauthor, *90 Minutes in Heaven*

"Boldly honest, marvelously comforting, and desperately needed. Yvonne Ortega clearly and unashamedly brings the struggles and, yes, the joys of surviving cancer to light."

Louise Bergmann DuMont, author, *Faith-Dipped Chocolate*

"Yvonne Ortega knows firsthand how frightening cancer is for any woman. She walks with you along the path of discovery through surgery and beyond, pointing you to God's help and hope in the midst of these valleys. She'll quickly become your friend as you discover you're not alone."

Lin Johnson, director, Write-to-Publish Conference; managing editor, *Church Libraries*

"Reading this book brought back all those complicated emotions I felt the year I was diagnosed and treated for cancer. Yvonne Ortega captures them all. If I'd had this book back then, I know it would have helped me. I recommend it to all facing their own journeys through cancer."

Amy Givler, MD, author, *Hope in the Face of Cancer*

"Ride the backward roller coaster with Yvonne as your seatmate on a courageous, vulnerable, hope-filled journey *through* cancer. You won't know whether to laugh or cry— but you will know you've found a friend."

Jane Rubietta, author, *Resting Place*

Finding Hope
for
Your Journey
through
Breast Cancer

60 Inspirational Readings

Yvonne Ortega

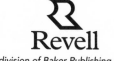

Revell
a division of Baker Publishing Group
Grand Rapids, Michigan

In loving memory of my cousin,
Theresa Shields,
who fought valiantly to the end
in her battle against cancer

———————————————

© 2007, 2010 by Yvonne Ortega

Published by Revell
a division of Baker Publishing Group
P.O. Box 6287, Grand Rapids, MI 49516-6287
www.revellbooks.com

Previously published in 2007 under the title *Hope for the Journey through Cancer*

Printed in the United States of America

Library of Congress Cataloging-in-Publication Data
Ortega, Yvonne, 1943–
    [Hope for the journey through cancer]
    Finding hope for your journey through breast cancer : 60 inspirational readings / Yvonne Ortega.
        p.   cm.
    "Previously published in 2006 under the title Hope for the journey through cancer"—T.p. verso.
    ISBN 978-0-8007-3409-1 (pbk.)
    1. Breast—Cancer—Patients—Prayers and devotions. 2. Ortega, Yvonne, 1943– I. Title.
BV4910.33.O78 2010
242'.4—dc22   2010013235

Unless otherwise indicated, Scripture is taken from the Holy Bible, New International Version®, NIV®. Copyright © 1973, 1978, 1984 by Biblica, Inc.™. Used by permission of Zondervan. All rights reserved worldwide. www.zondervan.com

Scripture marked KJV is taken from the King James Version of the Bible.

10   11   12   13   14   15   16   7 6 5 4 3 2 1

Contents

Part Three: Treatment

Acknowledgments

Many people helped me and prayed for me along the way. I thank God for all of them.

Lin Johnson of WordPro Communications and the Write-to-Publish Writers Conference saw the potential for this book, and she kept me on task at the American Christian Writers Mentoring Clinic in Nashville.

Dennis Hensley suggested I submit two or three of my cancer devotions to *The Secret Place*, so I did, and they were published.

Members of the Richmond Christians Who Write (RCWW) encouraged me at the monthly meetings and prayed for me, especially Coleen Kenny and Patrice Jones. Barbara Baranowski, an RCWW member, graciously edited my manuscript.

Debby Bissette, Donna Hines, Karen Schlender, and Arleta Turnbull gave me their input as cancer survivors. Glenda Brost and Carolyn Griffith expressed their viewpoints as family members of cancer patients.

My online writers group—Shirley Corder, Ruth Dell, Jan Kerns, and Elaine Heys—critiqued part of my project and prayed for a publisher.

Louise DuMont, Cecil "Cec" Murphey, and Susan Titus Osborn helped me with my book proposal and told me there was a publisher out there for my book.

Bill Petersen gave me the good news—a contract. Nan Snipes proofread my devotional. Lonnie Hull DuPont and Jessica Miles, my editors at Revell, assisted me in the process from manuscript to published book.

My Sunday school class prayed, then, when I received my contract, they took me to lunch and presented me with a dozen roses.

My parents have been my cheerleaders in this project from start to finish. I couldn't ask for more supportive parents.

To God be the glory.

Introduction

In 2001, I joined the ranks of more than one million people in the United States who were diagnosed with cancer that year. Their lives would never be the same. Neither would mine.

I was one of those women out of every seven or eight who are diagnosed with breast cancer sometime in her life.

As I would learn, women respond to cancer in at least four ways. The first response is denial. The woman in denial says, "Everything is fine." She denies or suppresses her thoughts and feelings. She may force herself to smile and laugh to keep from disappointing her relatives, friends, and church family. She may repress her thoughts and feelings because she believes others will think less of her. Perhaps she struggles to accept her human limitations. She has always met the needs of others and ignored her own. She wonders what people will do if she's not available. She tells herself that if she cries, she might not be able to stop. She refuses to frown or shed a tear since she fears that would ruin her testimony.

The woman in denial smiles on the outside while her heart breaks on the inside. She may wear bright colors to convince others she feels happy. She whistles or sings hymns when she would rather scream or sob. She has lived in denial for so long that she doesn't know what she thinks or feels anymore. She asks others what prayer requests they have, but she doesn't share her own. When complications arise, she pretends they don't exist. She thinks the world is full of joy, and she has to continue to spread sunshine.

The second response to cancer is negativity. The negative woman says, "I'm going to die." Everything seems threatening to the negative woman. She walks around in despair. She anticipates her imminent death from this disease. The slightest pain means the surgeon didn't remove all the cancer, and it has spread to her vital organs. She thinks that the medical oncologist doesn't understand how sick she gets from an aspirin, much less from chemotherapy. The radiation oncologist will surely burn her. The thought of going to the hospital terrifies her. She has heard all about staph infections, and she worries she'll get one and die. She writes or updates her will. She may even schedule appointments with funeral directors to compare coffins and prices. She must talk to the pastor and may set up her funeral service. She is unable to smile, much less laugh. She fears that surgery and treatment will be ineffective. Instead of praying, she cries and endures sleepless nights.

Family and friends try to offer support. But as far as the negative woman is concerned, they don't understand and therefore can't help her. This woman may resign from her job since she thinks she won't need the money any longer. She may give away clothes and possessions and write farewell letters. Hobbies and interests no longer appeal to her. She stares in the mirror daily for signs of physical deterioration. She may refuse to answer the phone or the door. Her Bible collects dust. "Funeral March" plays repeatedly in her head. Life has come to an end for her.

Anger is the third response. The angry woman says, "God, why are you doing this to me?" She lashes out not only at God but also at family, friends, her dog, and anyone else who crosses her path. She may be in a rage against herself, her genes, her family, the Food and Drug Administration, and the Environmental Control Board. How could God take her in the prime of life? Why didn't God give her better genes? Why didn't she take better care of herself? How could the government approve drugs that would increase her chances of getting breast cancer? How dare anyone smoke around her? Why did she waste her money on retirement and on plans for her later years?

The fourth response to cancer is hope. The hopeful woman says, "God, I know you are with me as I go through this." She pours her heart out to the Lord, admits she is riding an emotional roller coaster, and trusts God to ride with her. Even with this healthy, mature attitude, she will still have the tendency to jump between negative and positive reactions. The woman with hope will find it easier to be honest with herself, God, and a select group of friends. Some days she will feel energetic and positive. Other days she won't even want to get out of bed. Either way, she admits her struggles to trust God and to understand the purpose of her disease and pain. She prays and asks others to pray for her. More than reciting a list of requests to God, she converses with him. She sits quietly in anticipation of his response.

She searches the Internet, libraries, and bookstores for current information on cancer, and she discusses the pros and cons of the issues surrounding it with God.

When fear weakens her spirit, the hopeful woman cries out to God to strengthen her. When anger raises her blood pressure and increases her heart rate, she asks her heavenly Father to calm her down. Although depression strikes without warning, she says to herself, *Today I feel lousy, but tomorrow I'll feel better.* Because she doesn't keep her depression a secret, it loses its hold on her. She also gives God a chance to lift her out of it. She fights cancer with the Lord's help. Daily Bible study brings comfort, reassurance, and confidence.

This type of woman handles a diagnosis of cancer in a superior manner. Most of us, even at our best, don't meet this ideal.

When I discovered the lump in my breast two weeks before Christmas, I was in denial. I confided in few people. I didn't want to ruin Christmas for my family or my students. I sang Christmas carols and participated in all the school festivities as if nothing were wrong. The Christian counseling center where I worked part time had a Christmas party; I smiled and exchanged gifts with the staff without a word about the possibility of having cancer. I was with Christian counselors, social workers, and psychologists—people trained to help those in crisis—but I suppressed my real thoughts and emotions. I didn't want to dampen the holiday spirit. But by keeping silent, I felt alone and scared.

Three days before Christmas, a friend drove me to the hospital for a surgical biopsy. Another picked me up hours later. At the time, I thought I was doing the right thing by not telling my family. Yet if my son or my parents had done that, I would have been upset and would have wanted to be there to offer support and encouragement. My denial made that Christmas a sad and lonely one.

At other times I responded with negativity. I feared imminent death. Having received a black belt in karate, I assumed I was a strong person, but the diagnosis of cancer left me shaking and clutching tissues. Wearing makeup was no longer important. Thankfully a co-worker called me up, probed about my depression, prayed for me, and helped lighten the burden. But still I floated from one response to another without warning.

One morning, a co-worker asked me how I felt. "I'm angry with God," I blurted before I had a chance to censor myself.

"Oh, no, Yvonne, you can't be angry with God."

"Well, I am anyway!" I said, and raced away from her.

I *was* angry at that time, and I needed to process the feeling, not deny it. I learned quickly which people I could be honest with and which ones would judge me or feel uncomfortable with my sharing. I struggled not to take it personally if someone was uneasy with my gut-level communication. Perhaps that person was uncomfortable with her own situation and wasn't able to relate at a deeper level. Most of all, I found people who listened and let me work through the emotions I felt.

Some people considered it their duty to tell me why I had cancer. I'm not sure why, but I think they felt they were comforting me or encouraging me. Perhaps they thought they were pointing out how I had failed God or failed to take care of myself. I had to remember that their theories were exactly that—theories, not fact. The only one who really knew the "why" was God.

Well-meaning folks told me about their aunt, grandma, cousin, friend, or neighbor who had cancer. Maybe they said the first words that came to their minds without realizing how they might affect me.

"My aunt had cancer," one person told me.

"How is she now?" I asked.

"She died. And you know, it's been eight years, and I still miss her."

I can't count the number of times I heard such responses. I never understood why people did that, and I had to learn not to listen. Yes, Aunt Ellen died, and yes, cousin Margaret lost the use of her left arm because the cancer spread. But I wasn't Ellen or Margaret.

Through the two cancer support groups I joined, I met several women who had survived cancer and were doing well five, ten, fifteen, or twenty years after their treatment. God used them to bless me, to remind me that he was the one in charge and that not everyone dies of cancer. God was still with me and comforted me.

Some days I experienced a gamut of emotions within a twenty-four-hour period. I wondered if anyone understood me. How could they? I didn't understand myself. I longed for a book that would address all those feelings within a context of Scripture and prayer.

I found more comfort in the Scriptures in those days than I ever had before. As I read God's precious promises, I took notes, and the Bible came alive. The people in Scripture were human beings with strengths and weaknesses like me; they weren't perfect. For the most part, they didn't pretend to be.

Through surgery, chemotherapy, and radiation, God never left my side. I realized he was real. He loved me. He was faithful. I was more than a cancer patient to him. I was his daughter. Since he is the King of Kings, I was his princess.

I played praise and worship music, recited Scripture, and made plans for the future. I kept a list of ideas for a party after my recovery. My prayer was that God would let me finish my residency in counseling and help me pass the state exam to become a licensed professional counselor. The party would be a celebration of life and licensure. One year later, I completed my residency, passed the state exam, and had my party.

❧❦

What about you? If you or someone you love has cancer, what are your strongest feelings as you read these words? Which of the four responses sounds most like you—denying, negative, angry, or hopeful?

You probably have questions; we all do. When we move into a new and unknown part of our lives, questions are certainly one of the things we struggle with. How will treatment affect my appearance? Will I still feel feminine if I go through chemotherapy and lose my hair, eyebrows, and eyelashes? Will my husband still find me desirable? How will my family and friends react to me? Will I survive?

Some of us feel as if our lives have gone out of control, and they have. We are no longer in charge of our lives,

although we never really were. Cancer has ruined our immediate plans. We have to put some things on hold. We're
forced to make other plans, but even in the worst of moments, God is with us.

Cancer can shake the foundation of our faith. One minute
we trust God, and the next we wonder if he knows what
he is doing. One day we read and meditate on God's Word
and claim his promises with confidence, and the next we
doubt his faithfulness. Many of us cry out, "My God, my
God, why have you forsaken me?" Hours later, calmness
returns and we can say, "With God, all things are possible."
We are on the spiritual journey of a lifetime.

You are about to embark on a sixty-day journey with
me as we look for hope in the midst of cancer. (Although
I envision this book as a sixty-day devotional, you should
read these devotions as you wish.) I call the Bible reading
for each day a *Hope Builder*. Your heavenly Father is a God of
hope. Jesus, the Wonderful Counselor and Prince of Peace,
waits to meet you in the pages of this book. He is the Great
Physician. Allow him to minister to you through the Bible
passages and selected verses.

Members of your family may be trying to cope with
feelings similar to yours. They want to say something,
but they don't know what to say. Perhaps they are scared
to share their feelings with you for fear of upsetting you.
This devotional is for them too. God loves your family,
and he longs to comfort every one of them.

For those of you with young children, select passages
from this book to read to them. Talk to them about your

cancer. Children have a tendency to blame themselves for anything that goes wrong. Be sure they understand that they didn't cause your cancer and they can't cure it. Share the Hope Builder and Bible verses with them. Pray the prayer at the end of the devotion with them. Because Jesus loves little children and always has time for them, he will console them. Maybe they could memorize the Bible verses with you, and you could discuss what they mean to each of you.

If your friends say they wish they could understand what you are going through, share this book with them. As part of the body of Christ, they can be used by God to help you through the journey.

Take a copy of the book to your church library. Others in your church who have cancer or have family members with cancer can walk the journey too.

Neighbors may also struggle to understand you, your disease, and your faith. It's okay to let them know you are a normal human being. Invite them to join you on this spiritual journey of hope.

If you work outside the home, share the devotional with your co-workers. Most of them want to be helpful. Those closest to you may experience many of the emotions you do. They also long to make sense of this frightening disease. Perhaps you could read the devotional with them each day at break time or lunch.

You will never have all the answers to your questions this side of heaven, but you can experience hope in the midst of cancer. God's Word is not only for the good days; it is also for the bad ones. You can experience life after a diagnosis of cancer, and it can be an abundant one. My prayer is that as you read this devotional, God will wrap his arms of love around you and give you hope. I pray you will get to know the Lord in a deeper, richer way. May you sense his presence more each day and grow in hope.

For maximum benefit, I suggest you try these methods:

1. Use a Bible you can mark. Underline or draw a circle around the Hope Builder passages. Record a date by them.
2. Write the verses on three-by-five, wire-bound, ruled index cards to carry in your pocket or purse.
3. Write the verses on Post-It notes to place on your bathroom mirror, on a kitchen cupboard, or on your desk.
4. If you have a computer at work or at home, use the Bible verses as a screen saver. Memorize the verses and meditate on them. Repeat them throughout the day and ask God to make them real in your life.
5. Buy a notebook or blank journal to record your thoughts and feelings as you read the devotional. As you talk to God and wait for his response, journal your prayers and his answers.
6. Purchase a doodle pad to draw pictures of your journey through this book. Children in the family may enjoy doing this with you.
7. If you are musically inclined, set some of the Bible passages or verses to music.

8. Make use of any drama talents you may have and write skits to act out your responses to the devotions.

9. If you belong to a cancer support group, read this devotional at your meetings. Each of you could discuss how God has spoken to you through the Hope Builder, Bible verses, anecdotes, and prayers.

PART ONE

Diagnosis

Getting the News

Handling Anger and Fear

Struggling with Depression

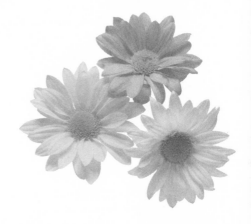

The News I Didn't Want to Hear

Hope Builder: Psalm 6:1–7

*Psalm 6:2–3: "Be merciful to me, LORD, for I am faint; O
LORD, heal me, for my bones are in agony. My soul is in
anguish. How long, O LORD, how long?"*

Hearing my surgeon say "malignant tumor," I felt myself
go limp. I stood in the teacher's lounge of the school where
I taught, holding the phone in my hand. My fellow teacher
and friend, Lucy, wrapped her loving arms around me and
began praying. I felt frail, and it really hit me that I was no
longer invincible and immortal.

It was lunchtime, but I couldn't eat. I left school and
drove to my second part-time job at the counseling center
to meet with my supervisor. On the way, I could hardly
see through the tears. I cried out to God, "Now can I be a
retreat speaker?" Somehow I thought that by going through
cancer, I would be paying my dues to become a retreat
speaker, which was my heart's desire. *God, I have only two*

thousand of my four thousand hours of residency in counseling completed. You called me to be a counselor. I've been obedient, and now you're going to let me die. I reminded him of the hundreds of hours I had studied and all the money I had spent on tuition and books.

When I arrived at work, my supervisor took one look at my face and seemed to know what the biopsy results were. He gathered the other staff members in his office to pray for me. I cried through most of that time. At one point I sobbed, "Oh, God, I'm scared!"

After meeting with my supervisor, I had no further appointments at the counseling center and left for the surgeon's office. My friend Pat met me there. In spite of her support and that of fellow co-workers, I felt indescribable anguish. No wonder the doctor told me to bring someone with me.

I returned home, vomited twice, and hyperventilated. I probably slept no more than two or three hours that night.

Receiving a diagnosis of cancer is a devastating experience. Our lives are never the same. We are not losing our minds. We are frightened, and this is natural. It's okay to cry. David cried. In Psalm 6, he said he was worn out from groaning and weeping all night long. If David, the man after God's own heart, could cry and ask for mercy, so can we.

Lord, be merciful to me, your child. I am so scared.
Keep me from fainting. Amen.

The Joy of the Lord

Hope Builder: Philippians 4:4–8

Nehemiah 8:10: "Do not grieve, for the joy of the LORD is your strength."

My friend Emily called me from Connecticut. She made a conference call with our mutual friend Stephanie in Pennsylvania. Em shared a beautiful Scripture with me and told me it was from Jeremiah 29:17. I opened my Bible and read, "I will send the sword, famine and plague against them and I will make them like poor figs that are so bad they cannot be eaten."

Em assured me she would find the correct reference. Not willing to give up, she quoted another uplifting Scripture for me and said it was 1 Samuel 25:19. I found the verse, but it was about a woman who hadn't told her husband something she had done.

Em then said the reference must be 2 Samuel 25:19, but 2 Samuel ends after chapter 24! Through all of this, the three of us laughed more than I thought possible.

I found I can still laugh at times. This morning I sang the song "The Joy of the Lord Is My Strength." When I reached the verse that has no other words except "Ha, ha, ha," I laughed through the tears.

We may wonder how anyone can laugh after a diagnosis of cancer. In Shakespeare's *Hamlet*, the gravediggers break the heavy mood by clowning around. In the TV series *M*A*S*H*, the military men laugh and joke when they are up to their elbows in mud and blood. Comic relief is a gift from God.

Perhaps something else is going on. When we are terrified, we can humbly bow before the Lord, read the Bible, and cling to every word.

In Philippians, Paul tells us to rejoice always and not to be anxious about anything. He says we are to think about what is lovely, excellent, and praiseworthy. So we can pray, sing, and laugh through the tears, or perhaps we may choose to dance before the Lord with tears in our eyes. Whatever we do, God promises us his peace.

Father, I thank you for a sense of humor and that the joy of the Lord is my strength. Help me rejoice in you, even when I am scared. May your peace guard my heart and mind. Amen.

Angry Thoughts

Hope Builder: Numbers 11:11–17

*Ephesians 4:26: "'In your anger do not sin': Do not let the sun
go down while you are still angry."*

*God, anger creeps in unannounced. You said you would make
up for the years the locusts have eaten. Is this cancer the way
you do it? If this is how you treat your children, no wonder you
have so few.*

I told my friend Carolyn about my feelings. She said
that life isn't fair. When I think about not letting the sun go
down on my anger, I wish it were daylight saving time. I
feel sorry for the people in Alaska since it gets dark early
there during the winter—they don't have much time to let
go of their anger before the sun goes down.

It's all right to be angry about having cancer. We don't
have to pretend to be perfect Christians who never have a
negative thought. Anger is one of the stages of grief. What
we do with it makes a difference. Talking to God about it

helps. He knows how we feel, but he wants to hear from us.

In the passage from Numbers, Moses was exasperated with the Israelites. He went straight to God and let him know it. God did not disown Moses for his honesty; he provided a solution for him. God told Moses to bring him seventy elders and then promised to "take of the Spirit" that was on Moses and "put the Spirit on them." They would help Moses so he wouldn't have to carry the burden alone. God doesn't want us to carry our burdens alone either.

Father, give me the courage not to let the sun go down on my anger. May I pour out my heart to you, as Moses did, and receive your answer. Amen.

Riding the
Roller Coaster Backward

Hope Builder: Romans 8:16–18

2 Corinthians 4:17: *"For our light and momentary troubles are achieving for us an eternal glory that far outweighs them all."*

What a lovely verse, but oh, how I struggle with it. Cancer is not a "light" trouble to me, and it seems like anything but "momentary." I cannot lie and say I'm feeling great. My insides would rip apart with the truth. Sometimes I don't even know myself anymore. I told my counseling supervisor, Marti, that I feel as if I'm riding the roller coaster backward; in other words, I feel powerless and scared.

As God's child, I am a coheir with Jesus Christ. But I find it easier to share in the blessings than in the sufferings. Who wants to suffer? Everything in me screams for relief. My knees shake so badly that it is not only difficult to see the big picture right now; it is also difficult to believe that there is one.

In life-threatening illnesses, we experience all kinds of emotions. We may feel as if the world we knew no longer exists, and we are right—it does not. For others to judge us or jam a pat answer down our throats will not help. God simply and tenderly offers us the Scriptures to help us deal with our emotions.

Heavenly Father, you are at work in my life and have
an eternal glory for me. Give me the strength and
courage to look at my circumstances in light of eternity
and trust you in this time of trouble. Amen.

The Red-Sea-Splitting God

Hope Builder: Psalm 18:4–6

Isaiah 43:2: "When you pass through the waters, I will be with you; and when you pass through the rivers, they will not sweep over you."

I called Mabel, one of my prayer warrior friends, to tell her about my cancer and ask for prayer. As she prayed for me, she referred to God as "the Red-Sea-splitting God." Tears came to my eyes as I thought about this powerful God who is my Father. I remembered Isaiah 43:2. I had once made a computer card for my son with this Scripture. Now I was the one who needed the verse.

Sometimes I feel the rivers raging over my head, and I'm afraid of drowning. Other times I see the waters as mountain streams, and God and I are walking through them together. I am barefooted and smiling. Whether I live or die, God is with me. He will not leave my side. The Israelites made it to the Promised Land, and I will make it too.

When we are seriously ill, we may feel that the torrents of death have overwhelmed us and are tossing us to unknown shores. We can call to the Lord and cry for help. He will hear us.

Gracious Father, I fear the cords of the grave are coiled around me. I know in my head you are the Red-Sea-splitting God, and the waters will not sweep over me. Help me know that in my heart. Amen.

Intended for Good

Hope Builder: Psalm 77:7–12

Genesis 50:20: *"You intended to harm me, but God intended it for good to accomplish what is now being done, the saving of many lives."*

Last night I visited a prison where I lead a men's domestic violence education and prevention group. I felt led to let the inmates know I would be out for two weeks for cancer surgery. I told one of the two chaplains about my diagnosis and requested five to ten minutes at the end of their service. With the chaplains' approval, I planned to combine my group with their chapel service to tell the men.

I fought tears and an uneasy stomach, but I managed to get through my group session. Afterward, God gave me the strength to be honest about my cancer. I quoted verses about all things working together for good for those who love God and are called according to his purpose, and about God not giving us more than we can handle. The substance abuse counselor sang a solo. We formed a circle, and the group prayed for me. One of the inmates quoted

2 Thessalonians 3:3: "But the Lord is faithful, and he will strengthen and protect you from the evil one."

The group sang the song "Sanctuary," and in vain, I tried to sing through the tears. Their prayers and singing blessed me, and I silently prayed for God to use my cancer to draw the inmates to him. I sensed divine confirmation when one of the inmates who hated women walked up to me, hugged me, and said, "I love you, Ms. Yvonne. It's going to be all right." He then brought my coat from the library and helped me put it on.

Joseph's time in prison was not wasted, and in God's economy, our time of surgery and treatment will not be wasted either. In the midst of our pain and terror, we can still touch lives for God.

We may wonder what good can come from having cancer. We may resent not being able to work full time or keep up with our church and community service. We may question where God is and why he is allowing this to happen. Doesn't he know we have family responsibilities? How can he interrupt our commitments? We can go to him with our questions and concerns. He will listen. He still loves us. He has not changed.

Heavenly Father, use my cancer for good in my life and in the lives of others. When I am overcome with fear and despair, may I remember your miracles not only in the Bible but also in the lives of those around me. Amen.

Tears and More Tears

Psalm 42:3: "My tears have been my food day and night, while men say to me all day long, 'Where is your God?'"

It was hard to tell my parents I had cancer. It was even more difficult to tell my son. We both cried over the phone. "Why do you have cancer, Mom? You don't drink or smoke. You eat right. You don't even drink coffee," he said.

All that was true, but I still had cancer.

I waited a week before telling the three of them. I kept telling myself I needed to process the reality of cancer and be able to talk without falling apart. I didn't fall apart, but I couldn't hold back the tears. *God, I know you're up there, but the tears still come.*

My "God is love" flag flies in front of my house, and I know God loves me, but I still cry at times. We can let the tears flow. God made us with tear ducts. In Job 16:16, Job said that his face was flushed from weeping, but God still

37

restored him. David, the man after God's own heart, said his tears were his food day and night. In Acts 20, when Paul told the Ephesians they would not see him again, they wept aloud, embraced him, and repeatedly kissed him. Paul did not judge them or push them away for their show of emotion. Even Jesus wept when his friend Lazarus died, although he knew he was going to raise Lazarus from the dead.

Crying does not make us any less Christian. God will not turn his back on us because we shed tears.

Father, you are the Lord who upholds all those who fall and lifts up all those who are bowed down. As I weep, comfort me, lift me up, and gently wipe away my tears. Amen.

Hit Broadside

Hope Builder: 2 Kings 6:11–17

Psalm 86:16: "Turn to me and have mercy on me; grant your strength to your servant."

My friend Phyllis, a board member from a local women's shelter, called and prayed for me, saying, "God, we know this did not hit you broadside." Immediately I remembered that Nancy, one of my prayer partners, had said, "Your cancer doesn't take God by surprise, Yvonne."

The cancer surprised me and hit me broadside, but not God. He is always ready to strengthen me. My part is to rest in his love and mercy.

In our darkest moments, we can cling to our loving Father. He is not the least bit shaken by our cancer. We may have a pounding heart and a swirling mind, or clammy hands and shaky knees. These reactions are normal, but we can draw on God's strength and shelter.

In the 2 Kings passage, Elisha's servant was terrified when he spied an army with horses and chariots surrounding the city. He concluded they were doomed. Elisha knew better. He prayed the Lord would open his servant's eyes. The Lord answered Elisha's prayer, and the servant saw the hills full of horses and chariots of fire all around Elisha.

Merciful Father, surround me with your horses and chariots of fire, as you did Elisha and his servant. Open my eyes that, like Elisha's servant, I may stand in awe at the sight of your divine protection. Amen.

The Blue Card

Hope Builder: 2 Kings 20:1-6

Psalm 61:1, 3: "Hear my cry, O God; listen to my prayer. . . .
For you have been my refuge, a strong tower against the
foe."

I shook from head to foot as I realized I had been praying
for myself and didn't even know it. For several years I had
kept a blue card with the names of everyone I knew who
had cancer. I had used it to pray that their suffering, treatment, and pain wouldn't be in vain. I prayed God would
use it for good in their lives and in the lives of others. I
asked that their cancer would be used for God's honor
and glory and for furthering his kingdom here on earth.
My requests were also for those who had cancer but had
not yet been diagnosed.

Now I added my name to the list. I sat outside on a
beautiful sunny day. The birds fluttered about and sang,
but I sobbed. *God, please make sense of this cancer for me. Please*

use it for good. Oh, God, don't let me die. I don't want my name crossed out as so many others on the card have been.

I want to live. My friend Dawn expressed it well when she said, "I want to grow old with my husband, sit on a rocker, and see my grandchildren."

You and I will experience similar thoughts and feelings. Unfortunately, we can all probably name relatives, friends, and neighbors who have died of cancer. Now we have cancer. We don't want to die any more than King Hezekiah did. He wept before the Lord, and God gave him an extra fifteen years to live. We also may weep before the Lord as he did and ask for more time on earth.

Abba Father, I come to you with the deepest cry of my heart, the desire to live. Be my refuge and strong tower against the foe of cancer with all its accompanying emotions. Amen.

PART TWO

Surgery

Surviving Surgery

Living with a Drain Bulb

Facing Chemotherapy and Radiation

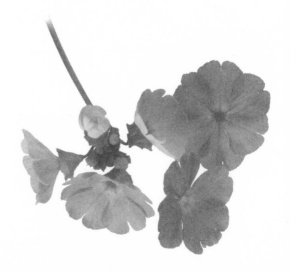

Memories of 1995

Hope Builder: Genesis 47:6–12

*Ephesians 6:2–3: "'Honor your father and mother'—which is
the first commandment with a promise—'that it may go
well with you and that you may enjoy long life on the
earth.'"*

Three days before Christmas in 1995, my dad received a
diagnosis of kidney cancer, and he underwent surgery in
January. I flew home to be with my parents for Christmas
and again for Dad's operation. Then, three days before
Christmas in 2000, I had a biopsy. In January my parents
were here for my cancer surgery to help take care of me.
How could this be? I'm the younger one; I should be taking care of them.

After their arrival, my parents and I went grocery shop-
ping. They wanted to stock the refrigerator with groceries
for my return home from the hospital. We had a delicious

Chinese dinner and would have gone to the mall, but I felt weary.

As I said good night to two teary-eyed parents, I whispered, "It's out of our hands now." Oh, how I hurt for them. *Dear God, please take care of them. Please comfort them. I'm more concerned about them than myself.*

Our parents' or other family members' terror and helplessness may break our hearts. We may worry about the strain and stress on our loved ones. But perhaps we can gain strength from the Hope Builder passage.

In the Old Testament, Joseph was second in command to Pharaoh in Egypt. After many trials, God blessed Joseph with the opportunity to provide the best land and food for his father and brothers. Perhaps cancer will be our trial before God blesses us in a similar fashion.

Heavenly Father, please meet the needs of my parents and other family members during the surgery and in all that lies ahead. May I honor them so all will go well with me and I may enjoy a long, abundant life on earth. Amen.

A Tenderhearted Nurse

Hope Builder: 2 Chronicles 28:15

Ephesians 4:32: "Be kind and compassionate to one another."

Two days before surgery, I filled out the preoperation admission papers and met Kathleen, a full-time nurse on the surgical ward who is a vibrant person. More importantly, she is a breast cancer survivor. Tears welled up in my eyes as I looked at her. *God, she's still here. Thank you.*

The morning of surgery, I experienced difficulty in the admissions office in my attempt to get my hospital bracelet, so I went to the surgical floor. Kathleen hugged me and told me she already had a bracelet for me. She also informed me that my surgery date was the one-year anniversary of hers. She said, "Next January 19, we will celebrate."

Oh, God, let me be here to do it.

Kathleen assured my parents and prayer warrior friends gathered in the waiting room that everything would be fine. As the orderlies wheeled me to surgery, she entered through the double doors to inform me that my friend Stella had arrived. I asked if I could please see her. Kathleen left and returned with Stella, who prayed over me and promised she would stay to pray with the others and keep my parents company. God reminded me through Kathleen and all those gathered to pray for me of how much he loves me.

As we go through surgery and treatment, God will bless us with some tenderhearted medical personnel and caregivers. It is his way of saying, "It's going to be okay. I haven't forgotten you. I know you need loving-kindness now more than ever. I will provide."

The men in the Hope Builder passage gave the prisoners clothes, sandals, food, drink, and healing balm. They mounted on donkeys those who were too weak to walk and returned all the prisoners to their fellow countrymen. The God who moved in the hearts of those men still moves in the hearts of people today.

Dear heavenly Father, sometimes I feel like a prisoner of cancer. As you provided for those prisoners in the Old Testament, provide for all of my needs. May I be kind and tenderhearted even as I struggle with this disease. Amen.

The One in Charge

Hope Builder: Romans 12:6–8

1 Corinthians 12:4: *"There are different kinds of gifts, but the same Spirit."*

I'm alive. I sighed in relief as I awoke in the recovery room. I felt my left breast. *Yes, it's still there. I've only had a lumpectomy.* Although my parents were in the room, the first person I saw was my friend Kandy. I laughed to myself and thought, *She probably told the surgeon what to do.* Then I saw Mom on my left and Dad on my right. Kandy said she let my parents go in the recovery room first, but I had my doubts about that. Whether the crowd is large or small, if Kandy is there, she takes charge. My dad lovingly refers to her as "the organizer."

Kandy's father had cancer twice. From that experience, Kandy knew I would want crushed ice to sip, and she searched the hospital floor until she found it. She told my dad to give me the crushed ice. Moments later, I turned my head to the right and opened my mouth. Kandy noticed my movements and told my dad, "She wants more ice."

We may laugh at this story, but we all can use someone with the gift of administration to advocate for us. I believe God will send people with different gifts our way as we need them.

We also have gifts from God. We may fear we can no longer be of service or that cancer has put us out of commission. The passage in Romans says to use the gifts we have. That Scripture places no restrictions on the gifts, such as only if we are in good health, at home, and able to drive.

Heavenly Father, in your mercy, give me an "organizer" on this journey. Show me how I can exercise the gifts you have given me, even though I am battling this illness. Amen.

Not Me!

Hope Builder: 2 Kings 5:1–13

*Matthew 11:29: "'Take my yoke upon you and learn from me,
for I am gentle and humble in heart, and you will find
rest for your souls.'"*

"You can't be alone the first week. You need someone there
day and night."

I cringed at these words from my surgeon. The thought
of needing a "baby-sitter" was humiliating to an independent person like me. I let him know I could manage by
myself. I felt like a two-year-old with my hands on my hips,
saying, "Me do it." I wanted to dash out of his office, but
my doctor told me he would keep me in the hospital for a
week after the surgery if I didn't follow orders. I nodded
reluctantly and left quietly.

When I returned home, I complained to my friend Carolyn, but she is a social worker. She immediately put her
professional skills to work and drew up a phone list, a chart

with shifts written in, and a meal calendar. She wrote her own name on the schedule and handed me the papers. My friend Kandy set up the shifts.

I was incapacitated after surgery and grateful for all the helpers who stayed with me. Friends from different churches and various denominations came and went around the clock. Surgery was a tough experience physically, emotionally, and spiritually, and I could not have survived the following week without those people.

Most of us see ourselves as strong, self-sufficient people. We don't want to hear a doctor telling us that we can't drive, that someone must accompany us on doctors' visits, and that we can't stay alone. We think, *That doctor doesn't know me. I can forget his advice and manage on my own.*

We may learn some lessons slowly. Our independent spirits may get in the way, but rest comes only in the acceptance of our limitations. God may shake his head, smile, and say, "My children, you will learn."

Loving Father, keep me from being like Naaman the leper. His preconceived notions about how he should be healed almost cost him his recovery. Thank you for my doctors and all those willing to help me in spite of my initial reluctance. Amen.

My Drain Bulb Angel

Hope Builder: 1 Kings 19:3–7

Matthew 6:8: *"'Your Father knows what you need before you ask him.'"*

I pinned a plastic drain bulb to my clothing, a visible reminder that the doctor had removed several lymph nodes during surgery. The drain or drainage tube was made of soft plastic. The doctor had placed it in the area of the incision to stop fluid from building up. He said the drain bulb would hold three or four ounces of fluid in a twenty-four-hour period, and when the amount decreased to one ounce or less, he would remove the bulb. When he told me I must empty and measure the blood from the drain bulb daily, I turned pale. My neck and shoulder muscles tightened.

"Doctor, I'm not the nurse type. I almost fainted when a neighbor showed me a boil on her arm."

He understood my fear and introduced me to Dawn, a cancer survivor. She offered to stop by each day and empty the drain bulb for me. I sighed with relief. She is a gift from heaven. With her daily visits, I'll also have reassurance of my progress.

It's all right to admit that the sight of blood nauseates us and to hope someone will help us. Not everyone will have a drain bulb, but we will all have some other concern.

In 1 Kings 19:3–7, Elijah was afraid and prayed he might die. God sent an angel to him with a cake of bread and a jar of water. The angel of the Lord returned to minister to Elijah and strengthened him for forty days and forty nights.

God sent both Elijah and me an angel. He is sensitive to our needs and will send us what is required.

Father, I take comfort in the fact you already know what my needs are before I ask. My requests are different from Elijah's, but they are real needs. Thank you for your provision. Amen.

Twelve Inches or Twelve Feet

Hope Builder: Psalm 31:24

Ecclesiastes 9:10: "Whatever your hand finds to do, do it with all your might."

Before I got into bed, I deliberately placed a mug of hot tea on the nightstand to the left of my bed. The surgeon had removed most of the lymph nodes on my left side; the drain bulb still in place reminded me of the pain. However, I was determined to regain full use of that arm. Getting into bed was challenging enough. My tea might as well have been twelve feet away instead of twelve inches.

The aroma of cinnamon apple filled the room. I looked at the mug longingly as I began the slow reach toward it. I groaned with pain, and tears came to my eyes when I picked up the prize. I warmed my hands with it and relished the moment before drinking the tea.

On this cancer journey, I am learning to be grateful for each small victory. As I move forward with the Lord, lessons in humility stare me in the face daily.

We don't all have lymph nodes removed, but if we have a life-threatening illness, we face struggles that those without one cannot even imagine. Jesus Christ is at the right hand of God making intercession for us, and the Holy Spirit "intercedes for us with groans that words cannot express" (Rom. 8:26). With their intercession, hope and determination can fill us to overflowing.

Gracious Father, give me strength to accomplish all the little things I used to take for granted. May I do with all my might what may be easy for others but is difficult for me. Amen.

Splashes of Joy

Hope Builder: Psalm 123:1–3

Psalm 34:5: "Those who look to him are radiant."

This morning I could finally take a bath again. I filled the tub with about two or three inches of water. After I struggled to get my nightgown off, I realized the drain bulb had to stay in place. I persisted with my plan anyway. I sat like a queen in a health spa, lacking only candlelight and music. The water refreshed my legs and feet. Since I couldn't get wet from the waist up, I held the drain bulb with one hand and washed with the other.

After my bath, I slowly plucked my eyebrows and put on makeup, dangle earrings, and perfume for the first time since the day before surgery. I looked in the mirror, smiled, and thought, *You look normal again, Yvonne. Thank you, God.*

I had a checkup at the doctor's office that day. I giggled at the thought of hiring the Goodyear Blimp to announce

I was clean, dressed up, and going to the surgery clinic, not to the surgery ward, this time.

We know we are making progress when we delight in getting ready for our debut after surgery. It's like old times again, or maybe better, because of what we've been through. We can look back at all that has happened and see the Lord beside us, full of mercy.

Dear heavenly Father, may I continue to look to you throughout my recovery. May I radiate your love and peace. Focus my eyes on you and show me your mercy over and over. Amen.

Not Alone

Hope Builder: Psalm 103:13

John 14:18: *"'I will not leave you as orphans; I will come to you.'"*

God's angels work in every hospital to comfort us. Marti is one of them. She is a survivor of breast cancer, not once but twice. She always smiles. An interesting array of bears, angels, cancer-awareness ribbons, and charms adorn her desk in the surgery clinic. Her personal lending library plus that of the surgery clinic help new and uninformed patients like me.

I remember the time Marti said, "There are worse things than breast cancer." My jaw dropped, and my brows arched in disbelief. I didn't believe her. Marti said we could live without a breast, but living without a leg or an arm would pose great difficulty.

God's angels volunteer in the community also. Since my surgery, my home has resembled a florist shop. My friends send me plants in every size in colorful pots to decorate nearly every room. They fill my mailbox daily with greeting cards and presents. I have more cards, gifts, flowers, meals, and visitors than I did for Christmas. Even without these items and the company, I am thankful to be alive. A teacher friend gave me a blank gratitude journal. Each day I fill at least one page, telling God how grateful I am for my life, the people in it, and what I can do for myself.

If we look around, we will see we are not alone. God would never think of abandoning us. When we put him to the test to see if he will keep his promise not to leave us as orphans, we can watch him pass it every time. If we keep a gratitude journal, we may have more to be thankful for than we thought possible.

Precious Lord, I thank you for being my heavenly Father and never leaving me as an orphan. Thank you for your compassion and for the people in my life who comfort me. May I cling to these Scripture promises and delight in how you care for me. Amen.

My Daily Carrot Juice

Hope Builder: Exodus 16:4, 11–15
Matthew 6:11: "'Give us today our daily bread.'"

Before my surgery, I could easily make fresh carrot juice. Now it presents one more challenge I cannot yet meet. Last week, my prayer partner, Nancy, brought me dinner and asked what she could do. I had run out of carrot juice, so I told her how to make it. We had fun together, and I was able to enjoy a fresh glass of carrot juice.

Nancy called again today to say she would stop by with a CD. She asked what she could do, and I asked her to make more carrot juice. God amazes me each time he meets my needs through those around me. He never sends someone early, but he never sends someone late either.

This recovery time takes us on a journey of faith. We will experience bouts of fear in taking care of ourselves, but we don't have to allow the fear free rein in our lives. We can give God a chance to meet our daily needs. God provided

manna and quail for the Israelites in the desert, and he will
provide for us in our desert of cancer.

> *Merciful Father, thank you for friends with servant*
> *hearts. Provide my daily bread in whatever creative*
> *way you choose. Thank you for the encouragement*
> *from the example of how you took care of the Israelites*
> *after their departure from Egypt. Amen.*

Love in the Storm

Hope Builder: Acts 27:37–28:2

1 John 3:18: *"Dear children, let us not love with words or tongue but with actions and in truth."*

I'm allergic to dust, mold, and mildew, so in the days before surgery, I would clean house every Friday afternoon. I miss being able to do familiar things like cleaning house and driving. My friend Carolyn cleaned my house for me before I came home from the hospital and again this weekend. She also picked up thank-you notes and sympathy cards for me. My friend is not *telling* me she loves me; she is showing me.

I appreciate my family, friends, and neighbors more each day. I wish I could jump out of bed and help them, but I can't. However, I can pray for them and ask God to bless them and multiply their time.

We may feel "shipwrecked" because of surgery or treatment. In the passage from Acts, Paul experienced a storm at sea that forced the 276 people aboard to abandon the ship. They all landed safely on an island, and the natives showed them extraordinary kindness.

I delight in reading today's Hope Builder. The same God who watched over Paul and the others loves us too. The people in our lives are "the natives" he provides to care for us on our island of cancer.

Abba Father, thank you for all those who love me not with words or tongue but with actions and in truth. Bless them and help me love others in the same unselfish way to the best of my ability. Amen.

Blood and Burns

Hope Builder: Psalm 3:5

*Proverbs 3:24: "When you lie down, you will not be afraid;
when you lie down, your sleep will be sweet."*

I woke up trembling, in a cold sweat, and with a pounding
heart. I checked my hands to see how bad the burns were
but couldn't detect a trace of damage. I sighed with relief;
it had been only a nightmare.

The previous night before going to bed, I had read about
chemotherapy and radiation. The saturated dressings on
my left side and the treatment literature brought on two
nightmares. In the first, my surgeon blamed me for the
excessive drainage. He told me I would have to find another doctor since we weren't a good match. In the next
nightmare, I went for radiation and didn't take off my
watch. I had burns on both hands and on my wrist under
the watch.

How I struggle at times to distinguish between my fears and reality. It is difficult but not impossible. After these nightmares, I literally placed my Bible on my overworked heart and went to sleep.

We may struggle to separate fact from fiction. We may be scared of the thought of cancer, chemotherapy, or radiation and have frightening dreams. We don't have to be stoic or robots at a time like this. The conflicts and emotions are normal reactions. God knows our frail nature, and he will sustain us.

Father God, I run to you to calm my racing heart. On my own, I am afraid. I ask you for sweet sleep. I thank you for each day I wake up. Amen.

Dracula's Blood Bank

Hope Builder: James 1:12

2 Timothy 2:12: "If we endure, we will also reign with him."

Saturday evening something warm and unexpected trickled down my left side. I checked the surgical dressing; it was saturated with bright red blood. My friend Carolyn changed the dressing for me and joked about being nurse Ratched from the movie *One Flew Over the Cuckoo's Nest.* Sunday morning she returned to do the job again. Two more changes by two other friends scared me into making arrangements to go to the surgery clinic the next morning.

Early Monday morning at the clinic, my surgeon asked me how I felt.

"I feel like Dracula's blood bank," I answered.

As my surgeon inserted a long needle in the area four times, the counselor in me studied his facial expressions and gestures to figure out what he might be thinking. Fear and anxiety swept over me, and I wondered what would be next. The surgeon ordered an immediate ultrasound and said he wanted to be there himself to view it. As he discussed performing surgery to remove the newly revealed clot, my knees shook and my stomach muscles tightened. *Oh, God, help me. Give my doctor wisdom and discernment. Don't let there be any more surgery, please.*

The doctor decided to wait on the surgery, and I felt relieved.

This journey turns and twists and tests our patience and stability. Nothing seems to go according to plan, but I am learning to gather every bit of my faith and keep going. The Hope Builder verse says God promises those who love him the crown of life once we have withstood the test.

God, give me a calm heart and a quiet spirit. I want to persevere under trial and receive the crown of life. My heart's desire is to place that crown at the feet of Jesus Christ and reign with him. Amen.

Clean at Last

Hope Builder: John 7:38

*Psalm 126:2: "Our mouths were filled with laughter, our
tongues with songs of joy."*

Water ran over me from head to foot. How luxurious. I
hadn't showered in eight days because of the surgical drain
bulb. With its removal, the water felt like a heavenly spray
over my entire body. I laughed and sang in the shower. My
friend Carolyn waited in the living room in case I needed
assistance. I did. With limited arm movement, putting on
my sweater became a two-woman task. But I was clean,
and I was making progress in my recovery from surgery.
I was also learning to be content with the simple things
in life. Showering and feeling refreshed were no longer a
given. Not much was.

When we face bath or shower limitations, we long for
the refreshment of soaking in the bathtub or standing in
a steady stream of water. In the meantime, we can find

consolation in today's Hope Builder passage. As a believer, more important waters flow from within.

> *Precious Lord, thank you for showers and all the simple things in life I previously took for granted. Fill my mouth with laughter and my tongue with singing for all I have. May I appreciate the streams of living water that flow from within me. Amen.*

A Mixed Message

Hope Builder: Psalm 71:20

Psalm 39:12: "Hear my prayer, O LORD, listen to my cry for help; be not deaf to my weeping."

"The good news is that there is no cancer in the lymph nodes."

I sighed with relief when I heard those words from my surgeon.

"But there is another cluster of cancer cells near one lymph node."

I was devastated, and tears gushed down my cheeks. *Oh, dear God, how much more?*

The doctor handed me a box of tissues. I thought I had shed all my tears during my separation and divorce, and then during my struggle with cancer thus far. Surely I had already filled the Atlantic Ocean once, if not twice. How could there be any tears left? My head throbbed, and I silently screamed, *God, I want to live!*

My doctor assured me it would be all right; six months from now I would look back on this and be glad it was behind me.

Oh, God, I can hardly wait. Let's fast forward through the next six months.

Our postoperative pathology report may not be what we want to hear. A cancer report can cause us more anguish than we thought possible and shake the foundation of our faith. Where do we turn? We can't help but be scared and sob. A normal reaction is to wonder where God is and if he has turned his back on us. We don't have to be afraid to ask him. He is God. He can handle our questions.

In today's Hope Builder, David says God made him see many bitter troubles, but he confidently proclaims God will restore his life and comfort him again. God's character never changes. Whether he restores us here or in the next life, God still comforts his children.

Abba Father, I come before you weak and weeping.
Console me, Lord. Bring a sense of normalcy to my
life and let me live. Amen.

A Swirling Mind

Hope Builder: Isaiah 28:29

Psalm 32:8: "I will instruct you and teach you in the way you should go; I will counsel you and watch over you."

Medical oncologist and *radiation oncologist* were once unknown terms to me. I wish they still were. Today my prayer partner, Nancy, and I went to the hospital to meet with both oncologists. While we waited, I noticed only elderly patients in the waiting room. Some used walkers; others sat in wheelchairs. Anger swept over me. "What am I doing here?" I whispered, and quietly pointed out the age difference to Nancy.

When the nurse called me by name, Nancy and I entered the medical oncologist's office and waited. As the doctor walked into the office, I cried and blurted out, "I'm so scared. I know God hears my prayers, but I wish I could *see* him."

The doctor hugged me. Then using a dry erase board, she carefully explained chemotherapy and answered our questions.

Next we went to the radiation oncologist, who discussed radiation therapy from start to finish. Overwhelmed with the magnitude of treatment, I became dizzy. I placed my head between my knees and asked Nancy to open the door. I didn't want to hear any more. I wanted to run and hide in the peace and safety of my home.

I left the hospital with enough literature from both doctors to start my own library. Somehow I will read the booklets and make a sound decision about what kind of treatment to have.

Seeing more than one specialist and trying to make an informed decision on my own frightens and exhausts me. Like the elderly patients leaning on their walkers, I am leaning hard on God's promise to instruct and teach me. I welcome his counsel.

Decision making is difficult in matters of life and death, and our minds swirl. Yet Isaiah 28:29 says that God is wonderful in counsel. We can claim that promise.

Heavenly Father, I pray I will be sensitive to your instruction and teaching. Thank you for counseling and watching over me. You are magnificent in wisdom, and I ask you to fill me to overflowing with that wisdom. Amen.

Longing for a Healing

Hope Builder: Hebrews 11:32–34

Matthew 9:22: "Jesus turned and saw her. 'Take heart,
daughter,' he said, 'your faith has healed you.' And the
woman was healed from that moment."

What a jolt of reality I had at a breast cancer support group meeting tonight. First a lady with short hair walked in, followed by a bald lady, and then a lady with the tiniest bit of hair. One young woman had had her first chemotherapy treatment that day and soon made an exit to vomit.

As the women talked and asked questions about the side effects of chemotherapy, such as sores in their mouths and problems with digestion, diarrhea, and constipation, I felt myself getting sick. My head throbbed, and my knees wobbled like Jell-O. Before long I sobbed, and someone passed me a box of tissues.

I noticed a table with Valentine's Day decorations and all kinds of refreshments in the hallway. How could anyone possibly eat Valentine's Day cookies and have a soft drink during this type of meeting? Why did I eat dinner earlier? I felt sick to my stomach. *Stop the merry-go-round. I want to get off.*

I wish I weren't going through this. I wish I could hide under a blanket, wake up, and have this behind me. I wish I were free of cancer or had healing power, but God alone has that power. His healing may be physical, or he may simply help me peacefully accept my circumstances. I'm convinced he knows which is better for me.

We all face similar struggles. We may think we're hanging on with only a shred of faith. It helps to remember that Gideon, David, Samson, the prophets, and many others were not born with an unshakable faith. Their faith grew day by day. Hebrews 11 says their weakness was turned to strength and they became powerful in battle. It's okay to admit we are scared, sick, weak, or powerless. God will meet us where we are.

> *Father, please tell me, "Daughter, your faith has made you whole." I also ask for emotional healing from the trauma of cancer. May I join the ranks of those who turned from weakness to strength through faith in you. Amen.*

Too Much Reality

Hope Builder: 2 Chronicles 13:13–18

Psalm 35:17: "O Lord, how long will you look on? Rescue my life from their ravages, my precious life from these lions."

My stomach knotted, I felt a lump in my throat, and my hands were clammy. I was watching a video about a patient going through surgery and treatment. The producer taped it live, and I felt myself becoming more and more upset. When the video was almost over, my friend Arleta called and asked how I was. I blurted out, "I'm scared, Arleta. I'm not doing chemotherapy." I told her about the video. "Well, don't watch it anymore, honey," she said.

Later that evening my mother called, and I also told her I wasn't undergoing chemotherapy. "It's your body," she replied. "Do whatever you want."

Cancer is overwhelming, and I want it to go away. I need a lot of prayer. I won't make it without the Lord's help. I thank God he doesn't have visiting hours, because I keep going to him with my pain and fear. He must be listening, because I'm able to sleep nights.

We may not all see the video I did, but we may still be scared. If we compared the horror stories we've heard about cancer and chemotherapy, we would probably drop dead from fear. Instead, let's be like the men of Judah in 2 Chronicles 13 and raise a war cry to the Lord. God heard the cry of Judah, and the people were victorious because they trusted in the Lord. He will hear our cry too.

Lord, spare me from the ravages of cancer and the lions of treatment. I ask for triumph in the battle against this disease. As there were 500,000 casualties in the enemy camp, let there be that many cancer cell casualties. Amen.

On the Road Again

Hope Builder: Daniel 6:27

Psalm 142:7: "Set me free from my prison, that I may praise your name."

I grabbed the car keys, laughed, and walked to the garage. For the first time in two weeks I started my car. I backed out of the driveway and felt like a new woman. I didn't go far—I went to a women's ministry meeting nearby—but I was driving, and that's what counted.

After the meeting, I decided to buy a few groceries. The minute I moved the grocery cart two feet, I knew I had exceeded my limits. I felt the life drain out of me. I was no longer walking but dragging one leg in front of the other. I leaned over the cart and begged God to help me finish quickly. One of the store employees who knew me asked if I was okay. I explained I had done too much in one day. She hugged me and told me to take care of myself.

I couldn't return home fast enough. When I did, my garage was a welcome sight. Only the strength of the Lord got me through the door and into my favorite rocker, where I collapsed for the evening. I received three phone calls and could hardly answer the phone, much less talk. In my desire to return to normal, I attempted more than I should have and paid for it.

Most of us have the desire to go on as before. We want to be free of limitations and be independent. Perhaps the work of God during this time of cancer is to mold us more into the image of Jesus Christ. Maybe the freedom comes in the acceptance of our present situation.

Heavenly Father, this cancer and its aftermath sometimes feel like a prison. Rescue me from my unrealistic expectations. Use this time to perform signs and wonders in my life, that I may be more like your Son and give you the glory. Amen.

Back to School

Hope Builder: Psalm 104:33

Psalm 23:5: "My cup overflows."

I practically bounced out of bed this morning to go back to work after two weeks of convalescence from surgery. It felt great to be in school again and be something other than an oncology patient. The kids never looked better. I had really missed them. Some of them ran up and hugged me. Others saw me down the hall and screamed, "I'm so glad you're back, Ms. Ortega!"

I did not realize what a privilege and blessing it is to work until I wasn't able to. I took so much for granted. I looked at all those eager, smiling students before me, and I silently thanked God for each one and for their prayers.

They couldn't do enough to help me in the classroom. When they saw me raise my left arm to write on the chalkboard, one student said, "Write lower, so it won't hurt your arm." Eating lunch with the teachers that day was special.

I knew I had missed everybody, but I hadn't realized how much.

This journey is not a solitary one. Many people, young and old, want to pray for me and encourage me. My cup does overflow, and I am thankful.

We will experience good and bad times during treatment, but compassionate, kind, and loving people will come alongside us and bless us. We may surprise ourselves by singing praises to God for our job, whether it is inside or outside the home, or doing other things we had never thought about before.

Dear heavenly Father, open my eyes that I may see the ways in which my cup overflows. I want to sing praises to you all my life for what I can do at home or at work. Amen.

To Life

Hope Builder: Genesis 12:1–4; 21:2–5

Psalm 118:17: "I will not die but live, and will proclaim what
the LORD has done."

Germany, prisons, schools, and shelters. At these words,
my eyes light up, my heart flutters, and I come alive with
the hope of being a retreat speaker in these places. As I
write this, I am gazing at a photo of me with two college
friends, Lois and Vicki. A friend took this picture at Lois's
graduation party over a year ago. Vicki had just completed
treatment for cancer. The three of us performed a creative
dance to a song entitled *To Life*.

Vicki called after my diagnosis. I cried as I told her about
wanting to be a retreat speaker.

"You'll be an even better one for having had cancer," she
replied. Then she told me she was leaving the next day to be
a speaker at a retreat. What an inspiration she is to me.

Perhaps many of us have a list of goals and dreams. We
may have sensed a call from God to a particular ministry,
a career change, or further schooling. We don't doubt that

we have heard from God, and others along the way have confirmed God's call on our lives. Now we are confused, disappointed, fearful, angry, or experiencing some other mix of emotions because of cancer, but we can still have dreams and plans. Cancer can disrupt them, but it need not destroy them. Perhaps Vicki is right; going through cancer may even make them better. I can think of half a dozen people who have survived cancer and are now praising God. They continue to follow God's plan for their lives.

In the Genesis passages for today, we read that God called Abraham and made a promise to him when Abraham was seventy-five years old. He was one hundred years old before he and Sarah had their promised son, Isaac. They may have gone from wondering *when* God would keep his word to *if* he would keep it. Sarah's efforts to take matters into her own hands instead of waiting on God's perfect timing reflect our tendency to question God or to rush ahead of him. As Abraham and Sarah gazed at the beautiful son God sent them, they knew the twenty-five years were worth the wait.

Merciful Father, let me live and joyfully proclaim
what you have done for me. Keep me from trying to
be your assistant administrator or executive secretary.
May I see the delays not as punishment or disaster but
as part of a better plan. Amen.

Strength in Weakness

Hope Builder: Psalm 81:1

Joel 3:10 (KJV): "Let the weak say, I am strong."

My heart raced miles ahead of my car. I was on the way to the prison to facilitate the men's group. I hadn't seen the inmates in three weeks. The correctional officers, the chaplain, and the substance abuse counselor greeted me with open arms. "I prayed and fasted for you, Ms. Yvonne," one of the inmates told me. Many of the other inmates said they had prayed for me as well.

An inmate from the chapel group had made an exquisite card for me. On the front of it were a cross, a soft red cloth, and the words "Ms. Yvonne." Above the cross, the card read, "There's healing in the name of Jesus." On the inside in calligraphy was Isaiah 53:5: "By his wounds we are healed." The inmates from both my men's group and the chapel had signed the card.

The chaplain asked me to speak to the men in the chapel and let them know how I was. When I walked in, they clapped. I smiled, raised one arm, and pointed toward heaven. The soreness in my arm, the fears, the doubts, and the sadness dissolved. God's grace met me in all my weakness and made me strong. What a gift.

On the way home, I followed the suggestion of Psalm 81:1 and sang for joy to God, my strength. I sang in praise and gratitude to him.

We may be weak and worn out from surgery or treatment. We sometimes wonder if we will ever be strong again. I found out that night that God is waiting to fill in the gap. His strength makes up for my weakness.

Almighty God, cancer makes me physically, emotionally, and spiritually weak at times. May I lean on you and say I am strong. Fill me with your strength that I may sing to you and "shout aloud to the God of Jacob!" (Ps. 81:1). Amen.

Surprise!

Hope Builder: Acts 28:11–15

Psalm 116:12: "How can I repay the LORD for all his goodness to me?"

"What do you mean, 'I can't go in the room'?"

A student stood guard in front of my classroom door. Although I knocked and asked the students to let me in, they ignored me. After ten minutes, they finally opened the door. They had tied three colorful balloons to my desk chair. The first balloon said, "You're so special"; the second, "To brighten your day"; and the third, "Hope you get well soon."

One student had baked a cake, frosted it with white icing, and written my name on it with pink icing. Another had made chocolate chip cookies. Others had lined up soft drinks and bright red matching plates, cups, and napkins on a table. They gave me a card they all had signed.

I burst into tears. I was momentarily speechless, a rarity for me. The students smiled and were proud of themselves for surprising me. My struggles with treatment decisions, limited arm motion, and endless visits to the hospital faded into the background. God blessed me through those students and once again showed me how much support I have. What precious teenagers God placed in my life. In the most difficult times, God was closer than I thought, and his little angels proved it.

As we read in today's Hope Builder passage, Paul arrived in Rome after several delays. Many believers had traveled a great distance to meet him there, and their presence encouraged Paul. He thanked God for them. Similarly, in the midst of our trials and tribulations, God will send us loving people to encourage us and give us hope.

Abba Father, I pray I will sense your closeness and kindness each day. Thank you for each person you send to comfort and support me. Help me pass this goodness on to others during the recovery journey. Amen.

The Poster Child for Cancer

Hope Builder: 2 Corinthians 12:7–10

Psalm 73:26: "My flesh and my heart may fail, but God is the strength of my heart and my portion forever."

I beamed from ear to ear as I held my left arm straight up in the air. I bent it over my head and reached for the tip of the opposite ear. I was delighted with my progress.

"You should be the poster child for cancer," my surgeon said, smiling.

Laughing, I remembered the day after surgery when my arm felt as heavy as a cement block. A week later, I had struggled to do rehabilitative exercises with a video; the excruciating pain had limited my mobility to one-fourth of what it is now.

At the end of the rehabilitative video, the instructor had said, "Let's review all the exercises." I couldn't believe it when she said to do them three times daily. I collapsed on the couch and moaned, "You can review them without me." She really expected me to go through that torture three times every day? I begged God to help me. I couldn't manage one round of those exercises daily, much less three, but I wanted to regain full use of my arm. I took hold of God's strength and hung in there.

Whether or not we have had lymph nodes removed, cancer brings all kinds of pain and difficulties. This journey tests our resources on a daily basis, but God is always near and loves to help his children.

In the Hope Builder passage, Paul didn't want the thorn in his side any more than we want cancer. God told Paul that his grace was sufficient and his power was made perfect in weakness. Paul could live with the thorn because God gave him the grace to do so.

Heavenly Father, my flesh and my heart often fail. Cancer is a thorn in my side. May your grace be sufficient for me, so I can say as Paul did, "When I am weak, then I am strong" (2 Cor. 12:10). Amen.

I Want to Live!

Hope Builder: Psalm 46:1–3

John 17:15: "'My prayer is not that you take them out of the
world but that you protect them from the evil one.'"

"The Armed Forces Institute of Pathology did a deeper cut
on the tissue. The cancer is adjacent to one lymph node,
but it is also in that lymph node."

I stared into my surgeon's eyes while he read the report
to me. My world came tumbling down again. *Oh, dear God,
I want to live. Please let me live.*

Our conversation moved from radiation to chemotherapy
followed by radiation. My fear turned to terror.

When I returned home from the doctor's office, my friend
Kandy called. I told her what the doctor had said and then
cried out, "I want to live! I want to live!"

We all have an expiration date, but we seldom think
about it. Those of us with a diagnosis of cancer begin to
consider it. Some of us fight to live. Others give up and

walk around with an attitude of gloom and doom. I choose to fight.

Even if cancer has not reached our lymph nodes, it is still enough to make our hearts skip a beat. We may feel as if the earth has given way and the mountains have fallen into the heart of the sea. Our thoughts may roar as the waters of the sea, and we may quake from head to foot like the mountains with their surging. These feelings are natural, but when we admit them to someone, their grip on us lessens. Furthermore, God longs to be our "ever-present help in trouble" (Ps. 46:1).

Heavenly Father, I agree with Jesus when he said his prayer is not that you take me out of the world, but that you protect me from the evil one. Please protect me from the desire of the enemy of my soul to discourage and destroy me. Amen.

PART THREE

Treatment

Making Decisions

Enduring Chemotherapy

Fighting the Fatigue of Radiation

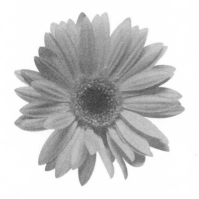

Decision Time

Hope Builder: Psalm 16:7

Proverbs 8:11: *"For wisdom is more precious than rubies, and
nothing you desire can compare with her."*

How I long for a few angels and trumpet blasts to confirm
my treatment decision. Will it be chemotherapy, radiation,
and tamoxifen (chemotherapy in pill form); radiation and
tamoxifen without chemotherapy; or an alternative ap-
proach? I have asked God daily for wisdom, searched the
Scriptures, asked others to pray for me, made lists of the
pros and cons, read the literature, looked on the Internet,
and talked with various people. I've watched videos advo-
cating both the traditional and alternative methods.

In my human frailty, I do not want chemotherapy, radiation, or tamoxifen. Reading a list of all the side effects of that
traditional treatment frightens me. The thought of foreign
matter in my body terrifies me. I prefer fresh vegetables,
fruits, bottled water, and herbal teas. An alternative ap-

proach sounds better to me; however, I wonder if any of the methods will heal me.

Two days in a row, I have awakened early in the morning. One of those times I woke up with nightmares about treatment. I was so scared that I couldn't even remember what the nightmares were about. I prayed, "Let this cup pass from me." Whatever I choose, I must walk in the will of God for my life.

The doctor gave me two weeks to make a decision. As the deadline approached, I asked God for confirmation. Someone offered to take me to the hospital for chemotherapy. One of my neighbors volunteered to spend the night with me. A professional colleague told me she would bring me dinner the day after chemotherapy. Two friends offered to flush daily my PICC (peripherally inserted central catheter) line, a device surgically inserted into a vein for putting chemotherapy into the body. Friends made those offers spontaneously, but I tried to convince myself they were coincidences.

Once again I could not sleep. Around 2:00 a.m., I knelt beside my bed and cried. I thought of Jesus in the Garden of Gethsemane, praying, "'Father, . . . everything is possible for you. Take this cup from me. Yet not what I will, but what you will'" (Mark 14:36).

I didn't want the cup either, but I couldn't fight God anymore. I told him he could have his way. If he wanted me to do both chemotherapy and radiation, I would surrender my will to his. Peace swept over me. I crawled back in bed and fell asleep.

As cancer patients, we face monumental decisions. Whatever we decide, we will live or die with the consequences.

I've learned to invite God into the process. I don't always like his answer, but I prefer to be in his will rather than out of it.

> *Heavenly Father, I need your wisdom as I choose
> a treatment plan. I do not trust my own wisdom,
> especially at this time. May I be attentive to your
> counsel and the times you instruct my heart at night.
> Amen.*

Struggling for a Normal Life

Hope Builder: Hebrews 10:23–25, 35–36

Hebrews 10:35: "So do not throw away your confidence; it will be richly rewarded."

"No, I cannot start chemotherapy that week. It would make me too sick to attend the women's ministry training in Virginia Beach. I would end up having treatment the Friday before Easter and wouldn't be able to eat Easter dinner. The other schedule allows me to be done the week before our women's retreat." I stood with my monthly planner before me while I talked on the phone with my nurse in the medical oncology clinic.

Cancer or no cancer, I am determined to go on living, to connect with people, and to confidently hang on to my dreams and goals. My medical oncologist wants me to stop teaching school during treatment, but I refuse. I will not stay home, dwell on this disease, feel sorry for myself, and get depressed. My health consists of more than the physical aspect. I'm an extrovert. I need to be with people. The compromise is that I'll have to wear a mask to work and continually wash my hands with antibacterial soap or wear examination gloves when handling student papers. The students said they prefer to have me in school with a mask and gloves on than out of school for a few months. Some offered to wear a mask themselves.

It is important for me to connect with others and to go on as usual to the best of my ability. I'm not ready to die, not even to my daily schedule. I will keep going to school and to the counseling center. I will continue to be a volunteer group facilitator at the prison.

How we struggle to connect and not give up. Sometimes we have to deal with those who want us to eliminate meaningful activities from our lives. In today's passage, Paul tells us to hang on to our hope and to encourage one another. He wants us to persevere and receive what God has promised us.

Merciful Father, I don't want to be so shaken by cancer that I stop living. Give me the grace not to throw away my confidence. Reward me richly. Amen.

My Strength and My Song

Hope Builder: Joshua 14:10–13

Isaiah 12:2: "Surely God is my salvation; I will trust and not be afraid. The LORD, the LORD, is my strength and my song; he has become my salvation."

What a schedule I endured at the hospital: first a scan to make sure my heart was healthy, then the surgical insertion of a PICC line for chemotherapy. My knees shook; my neck and shoulder muscles ached. I felt scared but reminded myself I could go through both procedures and still change my mind. I had the option to decide against chemotherapy at any time.

I had dragged myself to the hospital for the scan. I fell asleep during the process, perhaps from a combination of exhaustion from worry and confidence in the Lord.

Afterward, I stopped to speak to the American Cancer Society hospital volunteer, who is appropriately named

Grace. She accompanied me to the clinic for an explanation on the insertion of a PICC line.

The minute I sat down with the nurse, tears gushed down my cheeks, and she handed me a tissue. She assured me I could leave at once or receive the information before going home. She also said I could return the next day or the day of the first chemotherapy treatment.

I stayed. After she explained the PICC line, I consented to the procedure and prayed. Grace left, and I entered the surgery room.

Cancer is our mountain, but we are not alone. We can climb it with God and with those in our cancer support group. Caleb's courage can inspire us. At eighty-five years of age, he was as strong and vigorous as the day Moses sent him out forty-five years earlier. He was victorious with the Lord.

Abba Father, I thank you that you are my strength and my song. Help me trust you as Caleb did and not be afraid. Let me see this mountain of cancer through your eyes and rest from the war of fear. Amen.

A Long Day at the Hospital

Hope Builder: Deuteronomy 7:9

Psalm 94:14: "For the LORD will not reject his people; he will never forsake his inheritance."

My teeth chattered, and I felt sure I was going to turn blue. "You need to put up a beach scene, so people can think of warm things," I cried out. I was in surgery under local anesthesia for the PICC line insertion.

The nurse played a tape of California beach songs and told me the spotlight would be our sun. We all laughed, and the doctor began the procedure.

Afterward I thought I could go home. However, the nurse had to teach me how to care for the PICC line and change the dressing on it. This information was almost more than my brain could absorb after a morning at work, the heart scan, and the PICC line orientation and insertion.

I still had to pick up all the supplies for the device. I must have been a sight trying to drag a bag of supplies almost as tall as I am and as big around as a barrel. After the bag tumbled over twice, a kind man with a dolly took it to the front door of the hospital, while I made one last stop at the pharmacy.

Relief was on the horizon. All I had to do was drive the car around and pick up the bag of supplies. Yet every level of the parking garage looked the same, and I had no idea where I had parked. Exhausted and frustrated, I walked around for thirty minutes before I found my car. My left knee was swelling, and my feet and back ached from all the walking. I didn't know whether to scream or cry.

As I wondered how many items I would have to remove from the bag in order to lift it, a young lady in military uniform put it in the back seat of my car. After six and a half long hours at the hospital, I finally headed home.

That day brought several compassionate people across my path. God showed me through each one that he will take care of me every step of the way. I am his daughter, and he will not forget me.

Nothing about cancer is simple or manageable alone, and God knows this. He looks with love upon his children. He knows we are frail and feel overwhelmed at times. We can remind him of his promise never to reject us; he is faithful and will keep it.

Dear Father, forgive me in my weakness when I forget that you are my God and I am your child. I take comfort in reading about your covenant of love to a thousand generations of those who love you and keep your commands. Amen.

Shopping for a Wig

Hope Builder: Psalm 27:7–9

Psalm 27:7: "Hear my voice when I call, O LORD; be merciful to me and answer me."

"Buy your wig right away before you ever start chemotherapy," my friend Arleta said. "That way when your hair falls out, you'll already have it."

I knew she was right. I took my insurance papers and drove to a shop that caters to cancer patients.

The minute I walked in the door, the reality of my disease set in again, and I cried. The saleslady put an arm around me and led me to the wig section in the back of the store. She had nothing in my hair color and not a single wig that appealed to me.

As we looked through wig catalogs, my back and neck muscles tightened, and my hands got clammy. I told the saleslady I couldn't pick a wig by looking at pictures. I also mentioned that my friend Dawn had purchased a wig at that shop, didn't like it, and never wore it. I wouldn't have my insurance company pay for something I wasn't going to wear. Furthermore, the sign in the store read POSITIVELY NO RETURNS, so I thought I should go elsewhere.

The saleslady said she would order two wigs in my hair color. She promised me one of them would be perfect. She also assured me that if I didn't like them, I didn't have to buy either one. On the way home, I prayed that somehow I would be the exception to the rule and my hair would not fall out.

The thought of losing my hair made me sad. I didn't want to be bald. I couldn't imagine going around with a shiny head the way some people do. I also didn't want to lose my eyebrows and eyelashes. I knew it wouldn't be forever, but it still hurt.

God knows our hearts are breaking. We can tell him. He won't crumble or fall off his throne. David calls God his helper and Savior. He is the same for us.

God, do not hide your face from me. Be merciful to me on this cancer journey as I face one loss after another. You have been my helper in the past; be my helper now. Amen.

An Extra Charge

Hope Builder: Genesis 8:1

Matthew 10:30: "'Even the very hairs of your head are all numbered.'"

Yesterday morning I saw something on my feet while I stood in the shower. I feared it might be a spider, so I jumped out, put on my glasses, and noticed my hair was falling out in clumps. I didn't blow-dry it for fear I would blow the rest off my head and go to work bald as a Buddhist monk.

As I made my bed, I found hair all over my pillow. With a lump in my throat and tears in my eyes, I faced hair all over the carpet and everything else in the house, proof that I would not be the exception to the side effects of chemotherapy. *God, please help me keep a sense of humor.*

Last night I went outside to brush what hair remained on my head. A friend of mine consoled me when she said the birds could use the hair that fell out for their nests. I still had a lot of hair, but with the slightest touch to my scalp, it came out.

Today I had an appointment with David, my massage therapist. I told him not to rub my head because my hair would fall out. After the massage, I was alone in the room putting on my coat. I looked at the table in horror—hair covered the sheets. I called David to tell him. He looked at me and said, "I'm going to have to charge you extra to vacuum the sheets."

Oh, God, thank you for this man who could make me laugh when I hurt.

On the way home, I remembered Matthew 10:30. I told God I could count the hairs on my head too. There weren't that many. I thanked God that my wig had arrived that morning and that I liked it.

We may lose our hair, our eyebrows, and our eyelashes from chemotherapy. The loss is painful. As we look in the mirror, we no longer recognize ourselves, and we may shed tears. It's all right to cry. God knows we hurt, and our families are probably crying with us. Our hair will grow back, and in the meantime, God will not forget us. God did not abandon Noah and the animals after they entered the ark. Neither will he abandon us. God sent a wind over the earth, and the waters receded for Noah. He will do no less for us.

Dear Father, no matter how bald I am, you love me and care about me. As you provided for Noah and the animals, provide for me now. Please send a wind over me and let the waters of cancer recede. Amen.

An Unexpected Setback

Hope Builder: Proverbs 16:9

2 Chronicles 32:7–8: *"Be strong and courageous. Do not be afraid or discouraged . . . for there is a greater power with us than with him. With him is only the arm of flesh, but with us is the LORD our God to help us and to fight our battles."*

Thursday I felt tired and weak when I sat at the dinner table. I leaned my cheek on my left hand and felt a tender spot under my jaw. By Friday morning my left cheek and jaw were swollen, and the mouth sores were worse. My medication and supplements were not working. Saturday I could barely open my mouth. My friend Dawn encouraged me to go to the emergency room, and my neighbor, Barbara, drove me there.

After the internist, the ear, nose, and throat specialist, the oncologist on call, and my oncologist conferred among themselves, they admitted me to the hospital. They said my blood counts were low, and the parotid (salivary) gland was infected.

I struggled with feelings of fear and dread—fear of the unknown and dread of missing work—and no longer being in control. Then I laughed at myself. I was never in control to begin with; I just thought I was. Discouragement had swept over me until I remembered the passage from 2 Chronicles. Satan can attempt to defeat me through the cancer treatment and its side effects, but God is with me. As a believer, I have his divine protection.

Disappointment and fear may rob us of our peace during illness. A setback in our treatment interferes with our plans. We may feel helpless and frustrated and weep before the Lord. However, we are still his children. We can lean on him and trust him to direct our steps.

Heavenly Father, may I face each setback with faith in you, for you are the one who fights my battles. Help me remember that no matter what my plans are, you direct my steps, and you do a better job than I do. Amen.

Bubbly Bob

Hope Builder: Isaiah 63:9

Psalm 71:21: "You will . . . comfort me once again."

A tall man with beautiful blue eyes and a wide, contagious smile paid me an unexpected visit in the hospital. He handed me a business card with the title "Medical Social Worker" printed below his name. Within minutes we were on common ground as we talked about the field of counseling and our mutual love of Mexico and history. We discussed the Mexican Revolution, which is a favorite with both of us. We laughed and talked as if we had known each other for years.

Then Bob and I discussed the suffering and pain of cancer and also the good that can come of it. I mentioned the cancer devotional I was working on and read one of the selections I'd written while in the hospital.

Bob asked about my goals after recovery and stressed the importance of having goals and dreams. My eyes sparkled as I told him about wanting to go to Germany, Scotland, England, and Israel, not only to travel but also to speak. We were soon talking about the Rhine River, castles, and other sights in Germany.

How grateful I was that the hospital realized the value of a medical social worker. The fears, the disappointments, and all the other concerns that come with cancer didn't seem overwhelming when I shared them with a person who could understand and encourage me. God used Bob to remind me he will comfort me.

Not all hospitals have a medical social worker. Perhaps we or our families can begin the campaign to get one. In or out of the hospital, a visitor who can listen and care about our feelings is a blessing from the Lord. As God faithfully showed love and mercy to his children in Israel, he will show love and mercy to us.

Loving Father, I thank you for the comfort you bring me through those who visit me. You lifted up and carried your children in the Old Testament. Please lift up me, your New Testament child, and carry me through cancer. Amen.

Freedom for the Captives

Hope Builder: 2 Corinthians 3:17–18

Isaiah 61:1: "He has sent me to bind up the brokenhearted, to proclaim freedom for the captives and release from darkness for the prisoners."

"It's Tuesday night, and I've been in the hospital since Saturday," I complained on the telephone to my friend Dawn. "I can't leave my room."

"I know it's not fun to be confined," she said.

"No, it's not, and they want an exact count of the number of glasses of water I drink. I have to urinate in a 'plastic hat' on the commode. Then they compare my fluid intake to my output. They even check my tray to see how much I've eaten."

"I know what you mean. I experienced similar struggles when I had cancer."

I continued with my tale of woe. "When I check my menu selections for the following day, I must write in lemon wedges and hard candies for the infected parotid gland. If I don't, the nurses will. They told me it helps to suck on them. They have me here like a hostage."

"They must be taking good care of you," Dawn said.

"Yeah, but this is America, the land of the free," I moaned. "I want to go home."

"I'll visit you tomorrow," she replied, laughing.

"I'll pack my things and be at the door so you can take me home."

She found this funny too, but I failed to see the humor in the situation.

After that call, I glanced at my Bible study entitled *Breaking Free* by Beth Moore. *God, if I can't be free physically, at least let me be free spiritually and emotionally.* I chuckled as I thought of my "great escape" plans with my uncooperative friend. Perhaps I can look at my hospital stay differently. God has given me time to spend in prayer and Bible study. I can fellowship with him and write more devotionals as he leads.

We don't welcome these hospital stays. They are not our first choice of activity, but we can make them a positive experience. Cancer makes us feel weak and helpless. Trapped in mortal bodies, we are captives of this disease, but the Lord can use these times to transform us into his likeness.

Dearest Father God, I'm scared and disappointed. Physically, I am a prisoner of this illness. Help me experience spiritual and emotional freedom and release from the darkness of cancer. Amen.

Reunions in the Hospital

Hope Builder: Proverbs 27:9

Proverbs 27:10: "Better a neighbor nearby than a brother far away."

"No one can touch me or hug me because of the low blood counts," I explained to my friends Bob and Arleta.

"I don't care what they say. I've got to hug you, honey." Arleta wrapped her arms around me as I smiled and welcomed her hug.

I was grateful for that Sunday visit from my longtime friends. Like every person who entered my room, they scrubbed their hands with antibacterial soap at the nurse's station and couldn't visit me without a mask if they had a cold or cough. Combined with my weak immune system, a cold or cough could threaten my well-being.

Bob anointed me with oil, and he and Arleta prayed for me. They cheered me up talking about mutual friends and their children.

Iris, one of my professional colleagues, lives within minutes of the hospital. She stopped by daily to see me and pray for me. We filled each other in on news about our teaching and families, and she gave me advice about taking care of myself.

My friend Pat is a newlywed who works at an office a few miles from the hospital. She walked in with the honeymooner's "glow." We hadn't seen each other in a month and had a chance to catch up on the events in each other's lives. She also offered me advice about not trying to do too much too soon.

My teacher friend Barbara came to the hospital with her two sons. The boys visited their sick friend on the same floor while she chatted with me. We talked more in one afternoon than we did in a week at work together. She brought me word puzzles and said she was glad the doctor had me resting.

At a hospital an hour from home, I didn't expect any company. All my relatives live out of state, but God blessed me with some special reunions. He reminded me through my friends that I'm not alone.

When we don't have family living in our area, we may worry about not having visitors, help, transportation, or godly counsel. Yet God says a neighbor who is near is better than a brother who is far away.

Loving Lord, thank you for those who are near. Bless my friends who come to see me at home or in the hospital during this difficult time. I appreciate their company, prayers, and encouragement. Amen.

Fight, Yvonne, Fight!

Hope Builder: 1 *Samuel* 23:14–15, 26–28

2 *Chronicles* 20:15: *"For the battle is not yours, but God's."*

For the third day in a row, my white blood count dropped. It was at 500 the day the doctor admitted me to the hospital. Normal is between 4,000 and 11,000. My parents called me daily. I had told them not to come, but now I was scared. Maybe I wouldn't go home for a long time. Maybe I wouldn't go home at all.

"You better get down here," I told my parents on the phone.

"Fight, Yvonne, fight!" my mother said, crying.

"I can't, Mom." I started crying too. "I don't have anything to fight with."

"You've got to fight," my mother pleaded.

"God will have to fight for me," I said as I recalled today's verse in 2 Chronicles. "It is his battle, not mine."

Cancer with or without chemotherapy is a difficult journey both physically and emotionally. We feel drained and don't have the strength to fight. We may fear we won't escape the complications of cancer. I thank God he is with us and fights for us.

In the Hope Builder passage, Saul pursued David to kill him. At one point, Saul and his forces were on one side of the mountain, and David and his men were on the other side, fleeing from Saul. David probably thought he was a dead man, but a messenger told Saul to return home because the Philistines were raiding the land. Saul departed and David escaped. God planned for David to be the next king. No one could take David's life and thwart God's work, and nothing can take our lives ahead of God's time for us. God may not use raiding enemies to save us from cancer, but he will take action to move forward with his plan.

Precious Father God, when circumstances seem hopeless, may I remember the battle is not mine but yours. I want to do what you have called me to do. Jesus, if I am to stay on this earth longer, intercede on my behalf and save my life. Amen.

Hopping with Hope

Hope Builder: Psalm 33:18–22

Romans 15:4: "For everything that was written in the past was written to teach us, so that through endurance and the encouragement of the Scriptures we might have hope."

I looked up from my hospital bed to see my friend Iris enter the room with several bags in her hands. She gave me notebook paper, two pens, two gallons of bottled water, and a magazine with an article about God's will for healing.

She still had one more bag. I squealed with delight as she brought out a card and an adorable white stuffed bunny with a lavender vest, a pink bow at the neck, and lavender on its paws and on its big, floppy ears. The bunny wore a pink turban, and so did I. (I had switched from wearing a wig to wearing a turban for ease and comfort during my hospital stay.)

Iris named the bunny *Esperanza*, which means "hope" in Spanish. One of the nurses put Esperanza at the foot of my bed. Whether reclining or sitting up, I could see my bunny.

I not only have Esperanza (Hope) with her cute little smile, but I have hope in God himself. This hospital stay is a test of my patience, but God teaches and comforts me through his precious Word.

In our fight against cancer, we face good days and bad ones. Sometimes we are optimistic, but other times we aren't. Today's Hope Builder says the eyes of the Lord are on those who hope in his unfailing love. We don't have to bear the burden ourselves.

Dearest Abba Father, thank you for the lessons you teach me during doctors' visits, treatments, and hospital stays. Bless me with the encouragement of the Scriptures so that no matter what happens, I will endure and not despair. Let your unfailing love rest upon me. Amen.

Out of the Cage

Hope Builder: Acts 12:5–11

Isaiah 55:12: *"You will go out in joy and be led forth in
peace; the mountains and hills will burst into song
before you, and all the trees of the field will clap their
hands."*

After my night nurse, Megen, listened to me read "Freedom for the Captives," the devotional I had written, she
wanted copies for all the cancer patients on the ward.
She invited me to type it at the computer. I sat straight
up in bed and smiled. Typing meant I could leave my
room. I had to wear a mask, but it was a small price to
pay. *Look out, world, here I come.* What a sight I must have
been with my hospital gown and robe, hospital slippers,
and a surgical mask.

My friend Iris was surprised when she visited and
found me at the computer. She sat next to me as I printed

two selections, and the fun started. Iris wanted to see a view of the Elizabeth River at night, so Megen took us to a floor with sliding glass doors overlooking the water. I breathed fresh air and stood at the threshold of freedom. Iris pointed out the Marriott Hotel, and Megen identified several tourist shops across the water. I mentally planned excursions to the hotel and the shops upon my release from the hospital. I could hardly wait to join the crowds again.

On the way back to my room, Iris and I commented about the beautiful murals on the walls. My nurse gave me permission to walk on our floor and see some of the others. I smiled and laughed with Iris as we strolled from one end of the floor to the other. We had fun trying to guess which national park, famous garden, or renowned historical building the artist had painted. We checked the information card by each painting to see if we were right.

I am slowly realizing I cannot take anything for granted. Life is precious, and the people God brings into my life, such as Megen, are special. Being able to walk from one room to another is a blessing. So is breathing fresh air.

Cancer may keep us homebound or in a hospital more days than we care to count. When we are confined to one room or to our home, we want to break loose and see something other than the same four walls.

Imagine the joy Peter felt when the Lord's angel set him free from prison in the passage from Acts. Initially Peter thought it was a vision, but then he realized the Lord had delivered him, and one way or another, the same Lord will deliver us too.

Gracious God, free me from the prison of cancer and let the chains of cancer fall off as the chains fell off Peter's wrists. May I go out in joy and be led forth in peace to sing with the mountains and the hills and clap my hands with the trees. Amen.

The Last Round

Hope Builder: 2 Samuel 22:32–33

Isaiah 40:29: "He gives strength to the weary and increases the power of the weak."

With both excitement and dread I went for my last treatment of chemotherapy. That evening, my friend Carolyn brought me a large pot of bright yellow Japanese daisies and blue Golden Anniversary flowers. She also gave me a colorful balloon with the word "Congratulations" on it. "You did it, Yvonne," she said, smiling. "You're done. Congratulations!"

I was done in more ways than one. I became sicker after the last treatment than ever before. As I hung over the commode, vomiting over and over again, I said to myself, "That's okay. This is the last time I'll be hugging this commode. I'll soon be well, and I'll be going to Maine in August."

I looked in the mirror to survey the damage. Except for a few strands, my hair had fallen out. My eyelashes and eyebrows had disappeared. My fingernails and some of my toenails were black, and the skin on my hands and feet had darkened. The medications to counteract the nausea and vomiting from chemotherapy made me sicker. I was worn out, and I looked as bad as I felt.

Cancer is a battle with or without chemotherapy. On our own, we have no strength or power, but we can cling to the promises of today's passages in the Hope Builder and in Isaiah.

Merciful Father, I am weary and weak from surgery and treatment. Arm me with your strength and fill me with your power. I trust you to make my way perfect. Amen.

Good-bye PICC Line

Hope Builder: Galatians 5:1

John 8:36: "'So if the Son sets you free, you will be free indeed.'"

I sailed across the bridge on my way to the hospital with excitement in my heart. It was time for the PICC line to come out. A nurse friend had said the risk of developing an infection or a blood clot increased the longer the PICC line stayed in my arm. That information settled it for me. Chemotherapy had ended a week ago, and I wanted to get rid of that thing as soon as possible.

Since my blood counts were satisfactory, the doctor gave her approval and the nurse removed the PICC line. I felt like a new person. Nothing dangled from my arm. I could shower without wrapping my arm in plastic to keep the PICC line dry. Rushing home from work to have a helper "flush" it for me would no longer be necessary. Weekly visits to the hospital for the nurse to change the dressing, flush the line to prevent blockages or infections, and change the injection cap would also end. My life improved in minutes, and I drove back home with a smile on my face and a song of thanksgiving on my lips.

This freedom is wonderful, but it pales in comparison to what we have in Jesus Christ. He came to deliver us from the bondage of sin and to give us eternal life with him in heaven.

We don't all have a PICC line or a chemotherapy port, but cancer changes our lives. Surgery and radiation restrict us for a while. Recovery from either removes limitations from our lives and gives us reason to celebrate.

How wonderful to know that the Son sets us free no matter what our circumstances. The yoke of cancer is temporary, but the yoke of slavery to sin is permanent without the Lord.

Gracious God, thank you that each step of recovery removes constraints from my life. Thank you also that your Son has set me free. Help me stand firm, especially during this time of cancer. Amen.

Germans and Muslims

Hope Builder: Psalm 66:16

Isaiah 50:4: "The Sovereign LORD has given me an instructed tongue, to know the word that sustains the weary. He wakens me morning by morning, wakens my ear to listen like one being taught."

Two weeks before the lumpectomy, I started seeing Sharon, a doctor of naturopathy. I continue to go to her for monthly consultations. Sharon always smiles and offers words of encouragement. She knows I want to be a retreat speaker and need to be strong, healthy, and energetic to do so.

Yesterday I went for a monthly checkup, and Sharon and I eagerly talked about the desire of my heart to go to Germany and minister there one day. Sharon had lived in Germany for seven years and was now getting ready for a visit there.

I told Sharon that God has given me a burden for the Muslims. She surprised me by saying many Muslim men work in Germany and send money back to their families. "Maybe we could go there together one day," she said.

My cancer led me to the person who wants to take me to the country God placed on my heart. I pray daily for the Germans and the Muslims and ask God to prepare me to teach them.

In the midst of cancer, God is at work. He brings people into our lives who encourage us and pray for us, and he teaches us through the most unlikely circumstances.

Dear heavenly Father, in or out of the hospital, living or dying, I hear your instruction. Wherever you lead me, may I be eager to tell others what you have done for me and to share the Word that sustains those who are weary. Amen.

Painted for Warfare

Hope Builder: Judges 7:12–21

Psalm 121:8: *"The LORD will watch over your coming and going both now and forevermore."*

I laughed as I counted all the red, purple, and black markings on my body. They extended from my throat to an area below my rib cage in preparation for thirty-three rounds of radiation. I looked like an Indian warrior from the old western movies, but my war wouldn't be against cowboys.

I would have to protect all those colorful markings and my entire body from the sun. I had to wear a scarf, long sleeves, and pants or a full-length dress or skirt during the hot months of May, June, and July, or else stay out of the sun. But I preferred this attire to the surgical mask and gloves I wore during chemotherapy.

As I thought about how I must have looked to others, I remembered Gideon and his three hundred soldiers. They carried trumpets and empty jars with torches inside. What a sight they must have been to their enemies, the Midianites and their allies, who were "thick as locusts." But the Midianites fled, and God gave their camp to Gideon and his men.

In our struggle against cancer, we are not alone any more than Gideon and his army were. At times we may feel abandoned and look ridiculous to others. These feelings are natural, and they do go away. Eventually we stop concentrating on externals and focus on our war against cancer.

> *Precious Lord, as Gideon triumphed over his enemies, may I triumph over the cancer cells that seem overwhelming. If you could use trumpets and empty jars holding torches for Gideon's victory, you can use radiation for my victory and force the cancer cells to leave my body. Amen.*

Giggles, Geniality, and George

Hope Builder: Proverbs 17:22

Job 8:21: "He will yet fill your mouth with laughter and your lips with shouts of joy."

To go over one hundred miles round trip each weekday for radiation seemed like more than I could bear, but my health insurance determined where I could go. Then I met George, my radiation therapist. He smiled from ear to ear and joked with me every time I went for treatment. When he laughed, his eyes sparkled. He teased me, and I teased him back. He told me some of his childhood adventures, such as the time he attempted to be Superman, went through the attic floor, and ended up in the hospital. God knew that chemotherapy had drained me and I needed more laughter in my life, so he gave me George.

With George administering the radiation, I could tolerate all the markings for treatment, the tape allergy, the skin ripped by tape, and the fatigue. I didn't expect to laugh my way through thirty-three rounds of radiation, but I did.

After we go through radiation, fatigue may set in. We may nap every chance we can, get up for dinner, and then sprawl on the couch for a few hours before going to bed. If we have had more than one surgery, chemotherapy, and other complications, we don't have much energy left. We may find it impossible to laugh. We may wonder if we will ever laugh again. These thoughts and feelings are part of the process, but with God's grace and the special people he brings into our lives, we don't have to be stuck with this mind-set. We can also find laughter again through joke books as well as comedies on television or from our local video/DVD stores or libraries.

Merciful Father, your Word says, "A cheerful heart is good medicine" (Prov. 17:22). I want that medicine. It sounds better than any other kind I've had. Amen.

Tangier Island

Hope Builder: Nehemiah 2:1–9

Psalm 103:1–2, 5: *"Praise the LORD, O my soul; all my inmost being, praise his holy name. Praise the LORD, O my soul, and forget not all his benefits . . . who satisfies your desires with good things so that your youth is renewed like the eagle's."*

With anxiety and fear of a negative response, I asked my doctor if I could have one day off from radiation. I told him I wanted to go with our ladies' ministry to Tangier Island on the Chesapeake Bay. I had never been there before, and the excursion would give me an opportunity to socialize with the women from my church.

The radiation oncologist smiled and agreed to let me go. I could hardly sleep the night before the outing. It would be a taste of a more normal life, and for the first time in weeks I would not have to go to the hospital for treatment.

The day of the trip, I wore a wide-brimmed hat, long pants, and a long-sleeved blouse to protect me from the sun. Once aboard the ferry to Tangier Island, I enjoyed the ride, feasted my eyes on the blue-tinted water and green trees, and talked with the ladies.

When we arrived at Tangier Island, I was like a little kid visiting all the shops. I toured the island on the awning-covered cart and ate a delicious family-style lunch.

On the way home, I couldn't keep my eyes open, but it had been wonderful to feel like one of the crowd out sightseeing, instead of a radiation patient.

For those of us who have been in treatment awhile, we long to be ordinary persons, to be able to do routine chores, and to have some recreation like other people. We may ask God whether our lives will ever be the way they were before. We may fear they won't be, but God's Word says that he satisfies our desires with good things.

This reminds us of the Hope Builder passage. Nehemiah asked the king for permission to travel to Jerusalem to rebuild the city and its walls. He found favor with the king and received letters for the governors to provide for his safe journey and for the keeper of the king's forest to give him timber. The time had come to rebuild the city. Nothing would prevent Nehemiah and the Israelites from accomplishing the task. Perhaps it is the same way with us: if it is God's will for us to recover, nothing will stand in the way.

*Gracious Father, help me remember all your
benefits. May I not only count my blessings but
also record them. As you helped Nehemiah rebuild
Jerusalem, help me rebuild my strength and my life.
Amen.*

Riding the Shuttle

Hope Builder: Psalm 68:19

2 Corinthians 2:14: "But thanks be to God, who always leads us in triumphal procession in Christ and through us spreads everywhere the fragrance of the knowledge of him."

For two weeks I drove back and forth to the hospital for radiation, but then exhaustion set in. I fought sleep on the way home. One day I nearly veered off the interstate. Startled and scared, I begged God to get me home safely.

The next morning at the clinic, I told another patient that I didn't know how I would last for another four and a half weeks of radiation. She told me I could take the shuttle from my area.

From then on I rode the shuttle. On the way to my radiation appointment, I would review my Bible memory verses. On the way back, I would sleep or think about God's faithfulness.

The stress of cancer can make us tired. Some days we may wonder how we will get out of bed, much less do anything else. Yet God will bear our burdens.

My friend Karen, who is a cancer survivor, says that in living or dying we can proclaim God's glory. She's right. Whatever the outcome, God can lead us in triumphal procession in Christ on this cancer journey, and we can spread the fragrance of the knowledge of Jesus Christ.

Dear loving Father, surgery and treatment bring me face-to-face with daily trials that I can't manage on my own. Thank you for bearing my burdens. Help me share your blessings with others each step of the way from earth to heaven. Amen.

Turbans and Tightwads

Hope Builder: Proverbs 16:16

Proverbs 16:20: *"Whoever gives heed to instruction prospers, and blessed is he who trusts in the LORD."*

With the heat and humidity of summer and my hair starting to grow back, my wig felt hot and heavy. I switched from wearing a wig to a lightweight pink turban, which cost me $19.95. Now I wanted a red turban and a denim one to match my summer outfits. Since I was teaching school only part time and had cut back on my counseling caseload during treatment, I struggled with spending so much money. I prayed and felt led to make my own turbans.

I found fabric on sale and made both turbans for less than half the cost of one. Even more exciting was the fact that I had the energy to shop for the fabric and to sew. I felt better and looked forward to wearing my new creations. God had helped me save more money and blessed me.

We may not all need a turban, but as oncology patients, we have other concerns. Perhaps we haven't thought of inviting God into decisions over little things, but God cares about every detail of our lives. Even with the best medical coverage, there are still many expenses. God longs to share his wisdom and riches with us.

Heavenly Father, without the gifts of your wisdom and understanding, my money won't stretch as far as it should. May I heed your instruction and prosper. Let me be among the blessed who trust in you. Amen.

PART FOUR

Recovery

Wanting the House in Order Again

Accepting God's Timing

Walking through the Doors God Opens

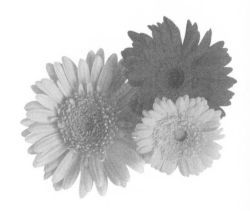

Getting Ready to Live

Hope Builder: Psalm 119:175

Psalm 91:16: *"With long life will I satisfy him and show him my salvation."*

I knew I felt better because the piles of clutter throughout my house started bothering me. For a week I attacked them one by one. First I went through the pile of cancer literature, bagged all the duplicate brochures and books, and took them to the hospital. I sighed with relief that they were no longer in my home and would be of service to others.

The second day I gathered all my get-well cards into a large red and white bag with hearts on it and put the bag in my closet. On another day, I found a place for all the candles, stationery, and other gifts from my family and friends. I worked like a soldier in preparation for a white-glove inspection.

I played praise music and sang to the Lord as I cleaned one mess after another. I repeatedly asked him to let me live so I could praise him. Then I thanked him as many times that he was granting my request.

As we progress in treatment, the disarray in our homes may begin to bother us. Perhaps some of us are not getting better, and it still annoys us. Others can straighten up our homes for us. Either way, we can praise the Lord. If God gives us a longer life on earth, it is for his honor and glory. If he takes us home, we will praise him with the angels.

Dear Lord, my heart's desire is that you will satisfy me with a long life on earth. However, if I am going home soon, help me be ready to praise you with the heavenly hosts and all the saints who have gone before me. Amen.

Fear of Lymphedema

Hope Builder: 2 Samuel 5:19–25

*Psalm 125:2: "As the mountains surround Jerusalem, so the
LORD surrounds his people both now and forevermore."*

"I got a compression sleeve before my flight to Italy. I couldn't
risk getting lymphedema." Those words from a friend at a
breast cancer support group rang in my head. My friend had
explained that a compression or lymphedema sleeve is used
to prevent lymphedema or an increase of it. It can be custom-
fitted or prefabricated and has varying degrees of elasticity.

During my biopsy, the surgeon had removed lymph
nodes and lymph vessels from my underarm area to see if
the cancer had spread. With the removal of both, it would
be more difficult for fluid in the arm to circulate to other
parts of the body. The excess fluid could build up and cause
swelling, thus leading to lymphedema. Radiation could
also increase the possibility.

Now concern set in. I had a plane ticket to my brother's
wedding and would have to endure three connecting flights.

I tried to get an appointment for a compression sleeve before the wedding, but the clinic had no openings for two months. I placed my name on the waiting list to no avail.

I prayed for wisdom. God led me to speak honestly with my family about the risk involved. After all I had been through, my parents and I agreed I should not travel without the compression sleeve.

As I looked at my new dress and my plane tickets, I felt disappointed and cried at my loss. I had been looking forward to the wedding and seeing my relatives, but I believed God would surround me with his love and comfort.

In the Hope Builder passage, David asked God if he should attack the Philistines. God told him to go, and he would give David the victory. When David faced the Philistines a second time, he inquired of the Lord again. God answered, but his battle plan didn't match David's. Yet David didn't try to alter God's plan; he obeyed it, and the Lord went before him.

When we have cancer, we face decisions, disappointments, and delays. They may not be the same as someone else's, but they still cause fear and frustration. God wants to comfort us and help us through the process. He can take our questions, no matter how many we have, and he will answer us.

Father, I want to get better, lead a normal life again,
and not be scared about the long-term effects of
cancer and treatment. As you gave David specific
instructions, please do the same for me. Amen.

In the Counseling Mode

Hope Builder: 2 Timothy 1:9

Isaiah 42:6–7: "'I, the LORD, have called you in righteousness; I will take hold of your hand. I will keep you and will make you to be a covenant for the people and a light for the Gentiles, to open eyes that are blind, to free captives from prison and to release from the dungeon those who sit in darkness.'"

I never thought I would look forward to returning to jail. I facilitate both men's and women's groups in their cell blocks. With chemotherapy behind me and school out for the summer, I picked up those two jail groups again. Meanwhile, one of my counseling supervisors and I worked on curricula related to domestic violence and anger management for clients who would be incarcerated, on probation, or on parole.

Then I went to a three-day retreat for jail-based personnel. As I listened to the speakers, God gave me a passion to work full time in a jail. I left the seminar knowing that when the job came, I would accept it.

After the retreat, I looked back on the opportunities God brought me in the midst of cancer. He allowed me to continue counseling and to add more hours to my residency. I reflected on the initial anger I felt toward God after a diagnosis of cancer. Reverence for the Lord kept me from lashing out at him, since he was the only one who could help me. God had called me to be a counselor, and it would happen in his time.

The Hope Builder passage says God has called us not because of what we have done but because of his own purpose and grace. Perhaps in our desire to rush through treatment and get on with our lives, we have stepped out with good motives but not in God's time or strength.

Merciful Father, I have been angry with you at times because of this cancer. I have also been afraid you won't let me live and fulfill your call on my life. Help me understand that you called me and you will accomplish your purpose in my life. Amen.

On the Farm at Last

Hope Builder: Isaiah 55:8–9

*1 Chronicles 4:10: "Oh, that you would bless me and enlarge
my territory!"*

Life with God is unpredictable and never boring. All
through college, I thought I would end up as a counselor
in a women's shelter. After graduation, I volunteered as a
group facilitator at a local men's prison for more than a year.
I found myself enjoying the group at the prison more and
more and praying that someday God would let me work
there. One month after my radiation treatment ended, the
supervisor of jail-based services called me for an interview.
My time had come, and I soon had a contract.

The prison is on a waterfront farm with cows, goats,
mares, peacocks, lots of trees, beautiful plants, flowers, and
birds. Sometimes before dinner, I run outside to stand by
the water at sunset. God strokes his paintbrush across the

149

sky and adds a breathtaking view to the sound of waves lapping against the shore and fish jumping in the water.

I am grateful to be a full-time counselor with co-workers who bless me daily. If I had not had cancer, I never would have had the courage to leave teaching and private-practice counseling. I enjoyed both, but I left with the certainty that I am in God's good, acceptable, and perfect will for me.

In his school of discipleship, God is teaching me to pray about the desires of my heart, to allow him to change those desires, and to trust him for his perfect plan and timing.

Perhaps in our illness, we all come to a crossroad in our lives. We may wonder what God would have us do. We may have a goal but sense that God has other ideas for us.

Dear heavenly Father, please enlarge my territory beyond my wildest dreams. Help me accept the fact that my thoughts and ways are not yours. May I recognize your timing and go when you open the door for me. Amen.

Lessons from the Trenches

Hope Builder: Philippians 4:11–13

Philippians 4:11: "I have learned to be content whatever the circumstances."

This past year has been one of the most difficult and terrifying of my life. I thought my faith in God was strong, but cancer tested it on a daily basis and revealed much room for growth. I had to accept my limitations, overcome my pride, and ask for help.

Living independently, I wanted everything in order and had cleaned house every week. I learned my house could go two or three weeks without being cleaned, and I wouldn't die of dust or clutter. I not only survived wearing a surgical mask and examination gloves to school, but I also realized they couldn't keep me from teaching and enjoying my students.

The outside world went on without me. My world turned with pain and sickness. Neighbors and stores changed their

flags and decorations each season, but the same flag I had
hung in December still hung in August. The basics of life
were challenge enough, but still each day was a gift, regard-
less of the season or holiday.

Before considering a full-time job in counseling, I had
wanted course work for state licensure out of the way,
residency completed, and license in hand. In fact, I had
preferred to keep teaching and counseling and have the
best of both professions. Instead, God pulled me out of
my comfort zone.

God wanted me to trust him and allow him to change
me as he saw fit. His plan was my peace, whether I was
living in ability or disability, whether I was teaching or
counseling.

We have preconceived ideas about our homes, families,
or jobs. It's human to feel fearful or dissatisfied when things
don't go our way, but the Bible says Christ gives us strength
for every situation.

*Gracious God, I pray I will be content no matter what
my circumstances. Help me trust you enough to believe
that good will come of my cancer here on earth and in
heaven. Amen.*

The Ultimate Healing

Hope Builder: Philippians 1:21–24

Philippians 1:21: *"For to me, to live is Christ and to die is gain."*

I'm not naive, and I'm not in denial. I don't believe everyone who prays for physical healing will be healed. I know not everyone who reads this book will survive cancer or the treatment. For example, I lost two cousins to breast cancer and other relatives and friends to all kinds of cancer. Their deaths had nothing to do with their faith or lack of it. They did not die because no one prayed and fasted for them or anointed them with oil.

We all die eventually. Some die sooner than others. Some die slowly, others quickly. Some leave this world with disease and pain; others slip away without any suffering.

I don't know why one person makes it through cancer and another doesn't. All I know is that God is still a God of love and mercy.

Perhaps when some of us get to heaven, God will say, "Welcome home, my child. I've missed you. I've waited for you. I couldn't bear to see you suffer any more." Maybe it is like my friend Glenda says: "God gives you the ultimate healing when he takes you home to heaven."

Whether we stay or go, we know this world is not our home. When we know Jesus, it is a temporary stop on the way to heaven.

It's okay to question the reason for our suffering, pain, and death. It's all right to wonder whether we should go to our heavenly home or stay on earth for the good of others. God can handle our conflict, and he does have an answer for us, even if it's not the answer we're looking for.

We may experience the same struggle Paul did. We love God and want to be with him, but we have not completed our ministry here on earth. We can say with Paul that continuing on earth will mean fruitful labor for us.

God, dying is eternal life with you in my permanent home. However, please grant the desire of my heart to continue living on earth for you and seeing others grow in faith and joy. Amen.

An Update from the Author

Much has happened since the first printing of this book. In 2004, Governor Warner appointed me to a four-year term on the Board of Counseling for the State of Virginia. On the way to Richmond for my first meeting, I realized there *is* life after aggressive cancer treatment.

I passed the state exam to become a Certified Substance Abuse Counselor and celebrated with a party. My parents, my two best cheerleaders, came to Virginia for the event. Two years later, I became a Licensed Substance Abuse Treatment Practitioner. That time, I celebrated by going to dinner with a prayer partner and other friends. As a cancer survivor, I've learned to commemorate every achievement and hope you will too.

Several times during the past nine years since the completion of cancer treatment, I've become apprehensive of aches and pains and wondered if the cancer had returned. This is a normal reaction for cancer survivors and one we will probably struggle with for the rest of our lives. Once I had a lump on my hip. *Was it cancer again?* My mind swirled with fears of a recurrence. I attempted to take deep breaths and relax. *Get on your knees and pray, Yvonne. Make an appointment with the doctor. Call a friend. Think about the false alarms you and your friends have endured.* I forced myself to do the things I would recommend that others do.

My primary care physician reacts the same way. During a recent bout with pneumonia, the X-ray was questionable because of my illness. However, the doctor didn't want to take any chances, "especially with your cancer history." I hate that phrase. You probably do too, if cancer is part of your life. A specialist eased my fears with the good news I didn't have lung cancer. My job and ministry would continue.

Throughout the Scriptures, God tells us scores of times not to be afraid. He knows we need constant reminders. He loves us and meets us in our panic over cancer, especially when we've been through it before. God understands when we imagine that every bruise, cough, or pain must be cancer again.

Certain things help me survive threats of recurrence. Initially, any time a new symptom appeared, I rushed to the doctor. Now I go for routine check-ups. I recite Bible verses, claim God's peace, and ask others to pray for me. I concentrate on my goals. I laugh every day, even at myself. Music fills my home. I count my blessings and worship the Lord. He is faithful to fill me with peace, and he wants to do the same for you.

I've traveled for TV interviews and speaking engagements from coast to coast to talk about God's love and faithfulness. He has honored my prayer to use cancer for good in my life and the lives of others. God can do that for you too.

A cancer support group provides us with encouragement, fun and fellowship. One of my cancer support groups still meets for dinner on special occasions, such as Christmas time and Valentine's Day. Our reunions remind us of how special life is. You can check with your local hospital or online for a support group near you.

Relay for Life continues to be the highlight of my year. Tears flow when an American Cancer Society (ACS) volunteer hands me my Relay for Life T-shirt, survivor pin and sash. As hundreds of us walk the survivors' lap, I thank God for the gift of life and all the family members, caregivers and friends who cheer for us on that first lap. You can call the American Cancer Society or check online at www. cancer.org for the nearest Relay for Life event in your area. If there isn't one, the ACS will help you start one.

In May of 2008, a cancer survivor friend and I flew to Vermont for the Stowe Weekend of Hope, a cancer survivors' retreat. I presented two workshops there. Cancer survivors, as well as caregivers, attended. I recommend this retreat.

I find it a joy to meet so many people who treasure each day and understand the emotional experience of cancer. If you live far from Vermont, you can ask your local hospital or support group to sponsor a cancer survivor's retreat in your community.

While I knew the complications of cancer or the possibility of a recurrence could change my plans at any time, I never imagined the losses I would endure after treatment.

In late 2008, one aunt passed away. Within weeks of each other in early 2009, another aunt died. My mother and my only child also passed away unexpectedly, none of them from cancer. I sobbed in anguish. After a struggle and many tears, my prayer was the same as during cancer. "God, use this for good in my life and the lives of others, for your honor and glory, and for furthering your kingdom here on earth." Bible study, prayer, Bible memory verses, praise and worship music, a support group, and a sense of humor helped me during treatment. They now help me in the grieving process.

Six weeks after my son's death, my father and I visited Alaska. We gazed in awe at hundreds of trees with green leaves, Mt. McKinley on a clear day, the glaciers, and the bears in Alaska. Never did I dream during treatment and after all those losses that I would enjoy life again so much. While in Alaska, I prayed about my future and discussed it with my father. The loss of family members, one after another, reminded me that God didn't promise me tomorrow. And once again, I felt led to make a significant change in my life. I realized God had not only called me to be a counselor but also to write and speak for him. I sensed he wanted me to counsel others on a wider scale, but I couldn't manage writing and speaking, as well as a full-time counseling job.

So on October 1, 2009, I began a new phase in my life as a full-time speaker and writer. I traveled to Ft. Rosecrans National Cemetery in San Diego, California, where my son's ashes are. Psalm 62:8 says, "Trust in him at all times, O people; pour out your hearts to him, for God is our refuge." At my son's graveside, I poured out my heart to God.

Before I left for California, God opened doors for me to speak for various ministries and at a women's retreat there. He reminded me cancer survivors can lead a full life and serve him after treatment and many losses. He does redeem our pain.

God continues to bless me. My father and I plan to visit Germany and Austria during the time of the world-renowned passion play in Oberammergau in June of 2010. By the time this book is published, we will—God willing—have shared in the sights and sounds of Germany and Austria.

As another outreach of my ministry, I send out a free weekly devotion in both English and Spanish via e-mail that will encourage you. If you would like to subscribe to it, please contact me at my website, www.yvonneortega.com. Be sure to indicate which language you prefer. My blogtalkradio show at www.blogtalkradio.com/hope-for-the-journey is on Tuesdays at 10:00 am to offer you further hope as a cancer patient/survivor.

If your church or organization would like to book me as a speaker, please contact me through my website. On the home page, you can download my one-sheet which lists many of the topics I speak on.

Please join me in thanking God for the precious gift of life. To God be the glory.

Yvonne Ortega is a cancer survivor, Bible teacher, freelance writer, and speaker who has also presented workshops on writing devotions all around the country. Her writing has appeared in many magazines, including *CBN.com*, *Spirit-Led Writer*, *The Secret Place*, *The Quiet Hour*, *The Virginia Alcoholism and Drug Abuse Counselors (VAADAC) View*, and other magazines, and she is a contributing writer to *The Embrace of a Father* (Bethany House, 2006). Yvonne received a literary award at the Maine Christian Writers Conference in 2002. She also received the Persistence Award at the American Christian Writers Conference in Virginia in 2002 for continuing to write during the time of aggressive treatment for cancer.